Transcranial Doppler Sonography

Edited by R. Aaslid

Springer-Verlag Wien New York

Rune Aaslid, Ph.D.
Director, Cardiovascular Research
Institute of Applied Physiology and Medicine
Seattle, Washington, U.S.A.

Product Liability: The publisher can give no guarantee for information about drug dosage and application thereof contained in this book. In every indivudual case the respective user must check its accuracy by consulting other pharmaceutical literature.

With 94 Figures

Library of Congress Cataloging-in-Publication Data. Transcranial Doppler sonography. Includes index. 1. Cerebrovascular disease—Diagnosis. 2. Transcranial Doppler ultrasonography. I. Aaslid, Rune. [DNLM: 1. Blood Flow Velocity. 2. Cerebrovascular Circulation. 3. Cerebrovascular Disorders—physiopathology. 4. Ultrasonic Diagnosis—methods. WL 355T7715.] RC388.5.T66. 1986. 616.8'107543. 86-22006

ISBN-13:978-3-211-81935-7 e-ISBN-13:978-3-7091-8864-4
DOI: 10.1007/978-3-7091-8864-4

Dedicated to E. A.

Foreword

Every few years a dissertation comes to the area of clinical application of medical technology which carries us forward as on a magic carpet into new regions of understanding and patient care. This book is such a magic carpet. It brings together, in a clear and incisive fashion, important hemodynamic principles with a simple noninvasive method of application to a part of the cerebral vasculature which has been relatively inaccessible. To the lucky and perceptive person who reads this book, a feeling of excitement and hope for progress is engendered. The diligent application of the potentials of transcranial Doppler ultrasound brings new power to our efforts in understanding the cerebral circulation and the causes, treatment and prevention of cerebrovascular disorders.

Merrill P. Spencer, M.D.
Director
Institute of Applied Physiology and Medicine
Seattle, Wash., July 1986

Acknowledgements

I am greatly indebted to Prof. Helge Nornes, Oslo, who introduced me to the fascinating study of cerebral hemodynamics in the early 1970's and since then continually encouraged my interest in this field. It was through his pioneering work on the cerebral circulation—using peroperative electromagnetic flowmetry and Doppler techniques—that the basis was laid for the noninvasive transcranial approach to the circle of Willis described in this book. I also gratefully acknowledge the stimulating case discussions with Prof. Peter Huber, Berne, at the very early introduction of transcranial Doppler, the inspiring exchange of ideas with Dr. Merrill P. Spencer, Seattle, during the last year, and the efforts of Dr. Alec Eden, Ueberlingen, to improve the English text on the subsequent pages.

Seattle, Wash., July 1986 Rune Aaslid

Contents

1. The Beginnings of Doppler

A. Eden

Whilst it is exciting to follow the current evolution of technology in medicine, a glance back in history to the scientific pioneers in this field is no less interesting and may help to maintain a sense of perspective as one new development appears to follow close on the heels of the last. In these pages it can only be a brief glance at three of the *dramatis personae* in this fascinating story, the main one being the Austrian physicist Christian Doppler, whose name has become a standard expression in noninvasive diagnostic methodology, but about whom so little is known as a person that a few biographical notes may not be amiss in the way of introduction.

On November 29th, 1803, the master stone-mason, Johann Evangialist Doppler and his wife Therese baptized their second son with the name Christian Andreas* in the church of St. Andrä in Salzburg just a few hours after his birth. The young lad grew up in the family house which still stands in Salzburg until the age of 19 when he was sent, on the advice of the mathematician Simon Stampfer, to the Polytechnic Institute in Vienna. After three years of what Doppler was later to call "a one-sided education" in mathematics and physics, he returned to Salzburg to complete his studies in science in 1828 and in philosophy the following year, both in record time. For the next four years (1829—1833) he was an assistant in higher mathematics under Joseph Hantschl at the Polytechnic Institute in Vienna, where he wrote in 1831, the first of his 51 scientific publications, entitled "A contribution to the theories of parallels". Like all of Doppler's early publications, it is of a purely mathematical nature, the works on physics appearing later.

The years 1833 to 1835 marked the low-point in Doppler's career. Despite numerous applications, he failed to obtain a teaching position and

---

* When a second given-name is used, Doppler is usually referred to as "Christian Johann" or sometimes "Johann Christian". The correct name, established by the author from the original records of baptism, seems not to have appeared in print until 1985 [7]!

worked for about one and a half years as a clerk in the cotton-spinning factory of Wachtl & Co. near Bruck on the River Leitha. At the age of almost 32, Doppler despaired of finding a suitable position in Europe and was planning to emigrate to the United States. He had sold most of his possessions and was applying to the U.S. Consul in Munich for a visa, when in 1835 he received offers from two institutes of learning. Doppler accepted the offer as Professor of Elementary Mathematics and Accounting at the State Secondary School in Prague, whilst rejecting an offer from Bern in Switzerland. (Had Doppler's choice favored Bern, it is interesting to speculate that this city—and not Prague—would have become the birthplace of the Doppler principle, as well as of transcranial Doppler 140 years later!)

Less than a year later Doppler obviously felt secure enough in his new employment to marry, on April 11th, 1836, Mathilda Sturm, also a native of Salzburg, who was to bear him five children. It was perhaps the additional obligations of matrimony and a family which led him to take over the additional post of Supplementary Professor of Higher Mathematics at the Technical Institute in Prague a year later. It has been suggested by contempories of Doppler [9] that it was during these years that he contracted the pulmonary tuberculosis from which he was to die. "His by no means very strong physique could not bear the strain of so many long hours of lectures in small rooms, overfilled with students", reported the Secretary-General of the Imperial Academy of Sciences during a special meeting in Vienna to honor their recently-departed member in 1853.

On 6th March 1841 he became a full Professor of Mathematics and Practical Geometry at the Technical Institute in Prague, and it was in this position that on May 25th, 1842 he presented the paper that was to make his name later famous, "On the colored light of the double stars and certain other stars of the heavens" before a meeting of the natural sciences section of the Royal Bohemian Society of Sciences in Prague, which was published in the proceedings of the Society the following year [3]. The contents of this paper and its effects on the scientific community in Europe at that time will be considered later in this chapter.

Doppler himself left Prague after some twelve years to become, on October 23rd, 1847, Professor of Mathematical Physics and Mechanics at the Mining Academy in Schemnitz, but the unrest that accompanied the Hungarian revolution forced Doppler to return to Vienna after less than two years. Here he became the successor of his old teacher, Simon Stampfer, as Professor of Practical Geometry at the Polytechnic Institute where he had started his academic career. By this time he had collected an impressive array of academic laurels. The Royal Bohemian Society of Sciences elected him to full membership in the year following the presentation of his paper there, he received an honorary doctorate from the University of Prague in

1847 and was elected a full member of the Academy of Sciences in Vienna in 1848.

It was 1850, however, that Professor Christian Doppler achieved the height of his academic ambitions. By a decree of the Emperor Franz Josef I of January 17th, he was appointed to the Chair of Experimental Physics at the University of Vienna and to be the first Director of the Institute of

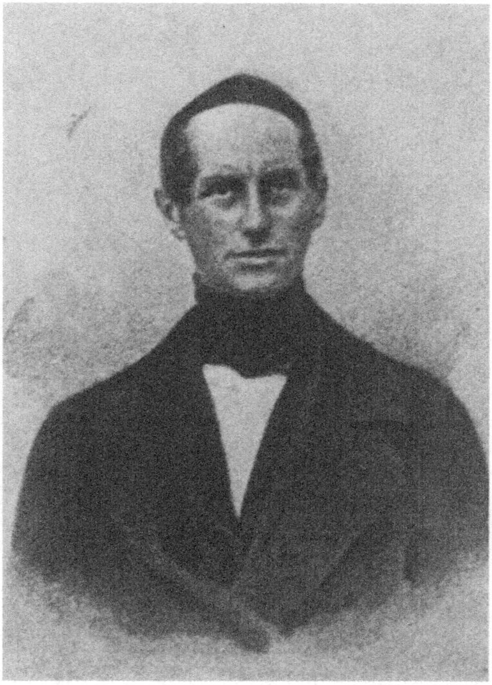

Fig. 1. This Daguerrotype is the only known photograph of Chistian Doppler. It is thought to have been taken in 1845 when Doppler was 41 years old and just three years after he presented his famous paper in Prague. It was discovered in 1904—in extremely poor condition—by Doppler's son Adolf, who had it restored. It appears here for the first time in the medical literature. (Reproduction by the author)

Physics which he was to found there. Among Doppler's pupils in Vienna was Gregor Mendel, the father of modern genetics, who studied physics there from 1851–1853.

Fate did not allow Doppler two years for the foundation of his new institute. Already in November 1852 he was compelled to take a holiday in Venice (which at the time was part of Austria) in the hopes of obtaining relief from his deteriorating pulmonary problems. He was accompanied by an old friend from his days in Prague, the philosopher and educational reformer Franz Exner, who was also suffering from tuberculosis and who was to outlive Doppler by only a few months. The mild climate of Venice did not provide the expected palliation. After five months illness, he died at 5 a.m. on March 17th, 1853 in the arms of his devoted wife, Mathilda, who had left their five small children in Vienna to be at his side during his last days. He was 49 years old at the time of his death in the Venetian Parish of

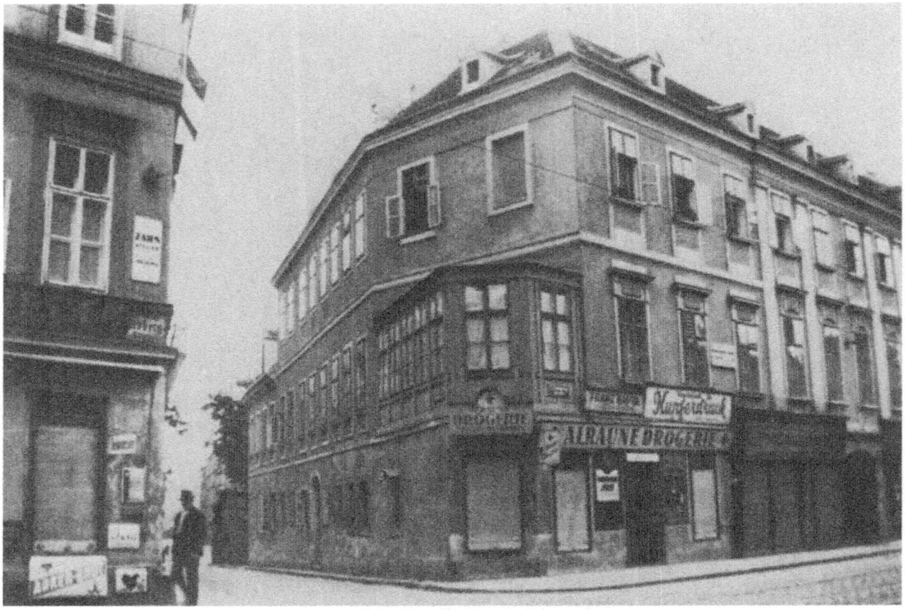

Fig. 2. The building in Vienna (Erdbergstrasse 15) in which Doppler rented the upper two floors for the newly-founded Institute of Physics. Doppler lived with his wife and five children on the upper floor. The building was badly damaged by bombs in the second world war and is now awaiting demolition to make way for an underground railway station. (Photograph by courtesy of the Picture Archives of the Austrian National Library)

San Giovanni in Bragora—the parish where the musican Antonio Vivaldi was born and baptized some 180 years earlier. We are told that the City of Venice provide him with "a grave of honor" and that the physicists of Venice erected a memorial to Doppler in the collonades of the cemetery. Although the author experienced little difficulty in tracking down Doppler's death certificate in the Venetian archives, all attempts to locate his grave have been unsuccessful, since records of burials were not made until Venice was reunited with Italy in 1861. Several thorough searches of the cemetery on the beautiful Island of San Michele have failed to reveal a gravestone. The memorial tablet in the collonades is now completely weather-beaten, with no legible word remaining.

The most valuable legacy we do possess of this "tall, lean man with glowing eyes, quiet and friendly but full with inner life, who lived only for science" [8] is undoubtedly his scientific work, but unfortunately very few clinicians, who use the Doppler effect daily, have ever read them—not even his *magnus opus* on the colored light of the double stars. This work bears the subtitle "An attempt at a general theory which includes Bradley's theorum

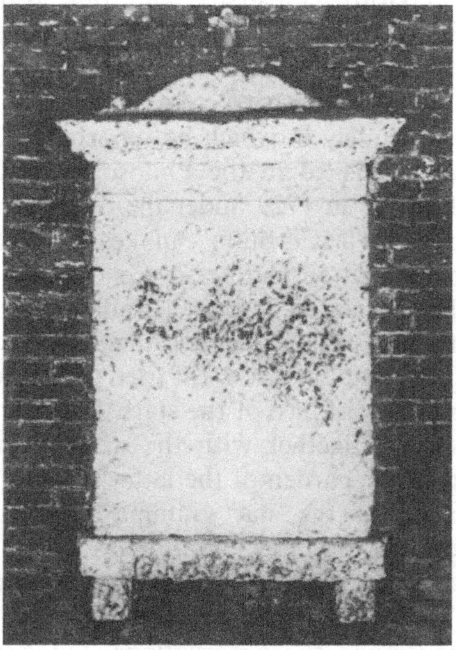

Fig. 3. All that remains of the memorial tablet, erected by the physicists of Venice at the time of Doppler's death in 1853, in the collonades of the cemetery on the island of San Michele. (Photograph by the author)

of aberration as an integral part". So, before considering what Doppler wrote, it is opportune to cast a glance back almost 120 years previously to the Englishman James Bradley and his theorum.

Bradley was born in Sherbourne, Gloucester, in March 1693 and was intended for the Church. The limitations of his father's income necessitated financial assistance for his education from his maternal uncle, James Pound, Rector of Wanstead in Essex and one of England's most noted amateur astronomers. The Reverend James Pound not only helped his nephew enter Balliol College, Oxford in 1711 for his theological studies (from where he received his. B.A. in 1714 and his M.A. in 1717) but he also encouraged his interests in astronomy. In 1716 Bradley was to make certain observations of Mars and nebulae at the request of the eminent astronomer—later Astronomer Royal—Edmund Halley, who was a friend of his uncle James.

It was Halley who one year later drew the attention of the Royal Society to Bradley's astronomical talent with the result that Bradley was elected a Fellow of the Royal Society in 1718.

The next year, 1719, Bradley was ordained as a priest and appointed Vicar of Bridstow, near Ross in Monmouthshire, but his career in the Church was short-lived—two years later he became the Savilian Professor of Astronomy at Oxford University and put aside all ideas of an ecclesiastical future. When Halley died in 1742, Bradley succeeded him as Astronomer Royal, an office he held with great distinction until his death twenty years later.

Bradley's letter to Halley in which he reports on the discovery of the aberration of light, published in the Philosophical Transactions of the Royal Society of London in 1729 under the title: "An Account of a new discovered Motion of the Fix'd Stars", makes delightful reading and is a fine example of how erudition and perseverence could transform an early fallacy into a brilliant scientific success. Bradley had been attempting to demonstrate the effect of parallax on the stars as the earth rotated around the sun. Robert Hooke had unsuccessful tried to measure this in 1669 as a basis for calculating the distance of the stars. Bradley erected a special 24 foot vertical telescope, together with the wealthy amateur astronomer Samuel Molyneux, in the garden of the latter's house at Kew, in order to measure the parallax of the star Gamma Draconis. They observed, however, a displacement too large and in the wrong direction to be due to parallax, and also found that other stars showed similar aberrations of position.

Molyneux discontinued the observations, but Bradley persevered in firstly checking the accuracy of his instrumentation and then making further measurements with a more conventional telescope. He tested numerous hypotheses to explain this phenomenon before correctly ascribing these aberrations as being to changes in the velocity of the earth in respect to the line of light from the star. "For I perceived, that, if Light was propogated in Time, the apparent Place of a fixt Object would not be the same when the Eye is at Rest, as when it is moving in any other Direction, than that of the Line passing through the Eye and Object;" wrote Bradley, "and that, when the Eye is moving in different Directions, the apparent Place of the Object would be different." In other words, the apparent position of a light-emitting object is dependant upon the velocity and direction of the observer in relation to the object. A recent reference to this observation as "the almost-Doppler principle" [6] is not as flippant as it at first might appear!

In his paper, Doppler frequently acknowledges "Bradley's perspicacious theorum of aberration" and his debt to this work. He commences by reviewing the wave theory of light, by which color perceived by the eye is dependant upon the frequency of the pulsation which stimulate it. Anything which changes the interval between these pulsations, changes the perceived color. If the light source and the observer are both at rest, then the observed frequency and the emitted frequency are the same. If the observer moves towards the source, however, the frequency will increase, and if he moves away it will decrease. Movement of the source will produce similar effects. Doppler used the analogy of a ship "which steers directly against the approaching waves and will, in the same time, meet a greater number and much stronger waves than a ship at rest, and even more so than one which moves along in the direction of the waves. Why cannot what applies to the waves of water also, with the necessary modifications, be accepted for the air and ether waves?"

After establishing a formula to the calculate the relative velocity of source and observer based on the change in frequency, Doppler takes an example from sound and calculates the velocity required to change the pitch of a note from C by a quarter tone. He continues: "A trained ear can recognize a change in tone at a speed of only a few—at the most 8—feet per second. However, I will now approach my real objectives insofar as I will immediately apply the above formulae to the appearances of light."

It is at this point that Doppler begins to get into deep water. He assumed that stars emitted only pure white light and was apparently ignorant of the evidence of infared and ultraviolet radiation which had been published forty years previously. He argued that the spectrum will be shifted towards blue if the source is approaching, and towards red if it is receding. He calculated that a velocity of 0.45 the speed of light would shift the radiation beyond the red end of the spectrum and it would become invisible. Conversely, stars that radiate outside of the visible spectrum would become visible if their speed relative to the observer changed sufficiently.

Based on this fallacy, Doppler then proceeds to give nine examples from astronomical observations—all incorrect—in support of his theory, including the influence of velocity on the color of both double and variable stars, the appearance of novae and the disappearance of the other stars. One should not lose sight of the fact, however, that although Doppler's paper was purely theoretical and unsupported by experimental work, and that none of the astronomical effects that he attributed to the Doppler shift were valid, his postulation of the Doppler principle and the illustration with sound were correct. His paper ends with a final reference to Bradley and his "brilliant explanation of the phenomenon of aberration. If a speed of 4.7 miles (sic) is sufficient to divert the direction of a beam of light by 20", then why should not a demonstrably greater velocity produce a change in color and intensity of the light?"

As was to be expected, the publication of Doppler's theory produced a number of scientific critics, and Doppler replied to some of these in learned journals. Indeed, his last publication before his fatal illness was to defend his theory against the mathematican Petzval, whose criticisms of Doppler's work were, in fact, due to a mathematical misunderstanding [5].

Certainly the most colorful critic was one Christoph Hendrik Diederik Buys Ballot, son of a Dutch reformed minister, and himself a lay preacher, who was 25 years old when Doppler read his famous paper in Prague, and who was working for his doctorate at the University of Utrecht which he was to receive two years later in 1844. Buys Ballot became Professor of Mathematics at the age of 30, and was Professor of Physics from 1867 until his retirement in 1888, two years before his death. He was the founder and first director of the famous Royal Netherlands Meteorological Institute, and is best known for the law concerning the deviation of wind which bears his name.

This young Dutchman did not believe that Doppler's theory could explain the colors of the double stars and decided to put it to the test. This he proclaimed in Latin at the beginning of a scientific work published in 1845 [2]. In those days there were no practical experimental conditions for attaining the high velocities required to test a suitable source of light, and even a similar experiment with sound waves was not easy. The maximum speed that could be achieved at that time was about 40 m.p.h. which was being reached by the new railways. Fortunately for Buys Ballot, the line between Amsterdam and Utrecht had been completed two years previously, and he was able to persuade the Dutch government to put this at his disposal, together with a locomotive and a flat-car, for his experiments.

For the first experiment in February 1845 Buys Ballot placed a horn player on the train and another on the side of the track. After calibrating their instruments, they both blew the same note as the locomotive passed the stationary horn player. Despite the noise of the locomotive and the interruptions caused by snow and hailstorms which resulted in the termination of the experiment, it was observed that the note blown on the train appeared to be almost half a note higher as the locomotive approached the stationary musician and half a note lower as the train receded. The experiments were recommenced in the more favorable weather of June the same year, this time on a more sophisticated scale, involving three teams of horn players and musically-trained observers, with Buys Ballot himself riding on the footplate of the locomotive. The results confirmed once again that Doppler's theory was correct—at least with sound. Experimental evidence as to its validity with light was not to be produced until the beginning of the 20th century by Belopolski.

In a paper commenting on the results of Buys Ballot, published in 1846 [4], Doppler was to conclude with the prophetic statement: "I still hold the trust—indeed, stronger than ever before—that in the course of time this theory will serve astronomers as a welcome help to probe the happenings of the universe, at times when they feel deserted by all other methods. The not insignificant interest that has already been shown in this theory, fills me with joyful confidence that the danger has passed for it to be put to one side, untested and unnoticed, perhaps to sink into oblivion".

The astronomical applications of the Doppler principle have been numerous. From the first rather crude measurement published by Sir William Huggins in 1868, who was able to demonstrate a Doppler shift to the red in the spectrum of Sirius equivalent to a recession of about 29 miles per second, a similar shift observed in nebulae is a major piece of evidence in the "big bang" theory of the expanding universe; measurement of the rotation of the sun and planets, and the variation in the rotation of the rings of Saturn which showed that they were not solid; and so on. Non-astronomical applications include the measurements of speed over the ground in aerial navigation, the tracking of satellites and the control of thermonuclear reactions. It enables the police to measure the speed of an approaching car, and it enabled Johannes Stark to demonstrate the effect that is named after him and for which he received the Nobel prize for physics in 1919.

This book is evidence—if evidence were needed—of the increasingly important applications of the Doppler effect in medicine.

References

1. Bradley J (1729) An account of a new discovered motion of the fixed stars. Phil Trans Roy Soc (London) 35: 637–661
2. Buys Ballot, CHD (1845) Akustische Versuche auf der Niederländischen Eisenbahn nebst gelegentlichen Bemerkungen zur Theorie des Hrn. Prof. Doppler. Pogg Ann 66: 321–351
3. Doppler C (1843) Über das farbige Licht der Dopplesterne und einiger anderer Gestirne des Himmels. Abhandl Königl Böhm Ges, Ser 2: 465–482
4. Doppler C (1846) Bemerkungen zu meiner Theorie des farbigen Lichtes der Doppelsterne ect., mit vorzüglicher Rücksicht auf die von Herrn Dr. Ballot zu Utrecht dagegen erhobenen Bedenken. Pogg Ann 68: 1–35
5. Doppler C (1852) Bemerkungen über die von Herrn Prof. Petzval gegen die Richtigkeit meiner Theorie vorgebrachten Einwendungen. Sitzungsber Akad Wiss (Wien) 9: 217–225
6. Eden A (1985) An early history of Doppler. Proceedings of the ultrasound diagnosis of cerebrovascular disease symposium, Institute of Applied Medicine and Physiology, Seattle
7. Eden A (1985) Johann Christian Doppler. Ultrasound Med Biol 11: 537–539
8. Poske F (1896) Johann Christian Doppler und das Dopplersche Prinzip. Zeitschr Physikal Chem Unterricht 5: 248–249
9. Die feierliche Sitzung 1853. Bericht des Generalsekretärs. Almanach Kaiserl Akad Wiss, Wien 1854

Author's address: Dr. A. Eden, EME GmbH, Postfach 1410, D-7770 Ueberlingen, Federal Republic of Germany.

2. Transmission of Ultrasound Through the Temporal Bone

P. Grolimund

Introduction

The problem of the acoustic properties of the skull were studied by White and co-workers (1967, 1978). The skull consists of three layers of bone influencing the ultrasound in different manners. The middle layer (diploe), has the most important effect on the attenuation and scattering of the ultrasound, especially when the bony spicules have a diameter comparable to the wave length. However, these spicules are absent in the temporal region where the skull is at its thinnest. The outer and inner table of ivory bone are important for refraction. The inner table follows the windings of the brain. This curvature will act as a lens and refraction can also be induced by these variations of thickness.

In this chapter the influence of the bone on the focused ultrasonic beam is discussed. Sections of human skull from the temporal region were investigated. To map the ultrasonic beam a hydrophone was used. The change of the beam profile and also the mean power, with and without skull sections, were measured and compared.

Material and Methods

Field Measurements

For ultrasound transmission, the same 2 MHz transducer was used as for clinical applications.The diameter of the piezoelectric disc was 16 mm. A polystyrol lens focused the ultrasound beam which was transmitted in a water tank. The walls of the tank were covered by ultrasound-absorbing material to avoid reflecting echoes. Above this tank, three screw threads were mounted, one perpendicular to the other (Fig. 1).

The hydrophone was fixed to a platform moved by the threads. Three step motors controlled by a computer were used to drive the screw threads.

The hydrophone was constructed by a 0.5 mm diameter disc of 10 MHz ceramic piezo material. Special care was taken to ensure the stability of the received signal. If the insulation was insufficient, measurements which take several hours were impossible. The received signal of the hydrophone remained constant for 2–4 days in water and no influence by humidity could be observed.

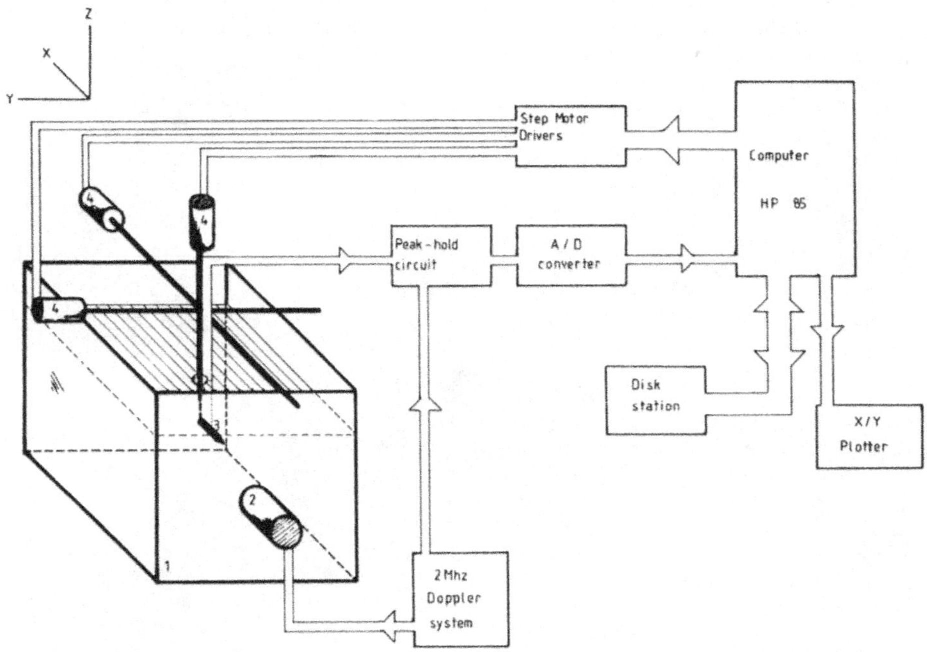

Fig. 1. Measuring system. *1* water tank, *2* transducer for US transmission, *3* hydrophone, *4* step motors

The signal received by the hydrophone went to an amplifier and analog peak detector. Next the signal was A/D-converted and stored in same computer controlling the step motors (Fig. 1).

The scanning pattern of the ultrasonic beam was the same during all experiments. First, the point of maximum sound pressure was estimated by moving the hydrophone. Then a further point on the transducer axis in the far field was taken to calculate the beam axis. The zero point of the Cartesian coordinates was the center of the transmitting transducer. This adjustment was made without a skull section in front of the transducer so that the refraction induced by the skull would be visible.

For lateral scans the starting point was chosen (20 mm = x and + 12 mm = y). Then the hydrophone was moved parallel to the y axis with steps of 0.25 mm to y = — 12 mm (97 steps).

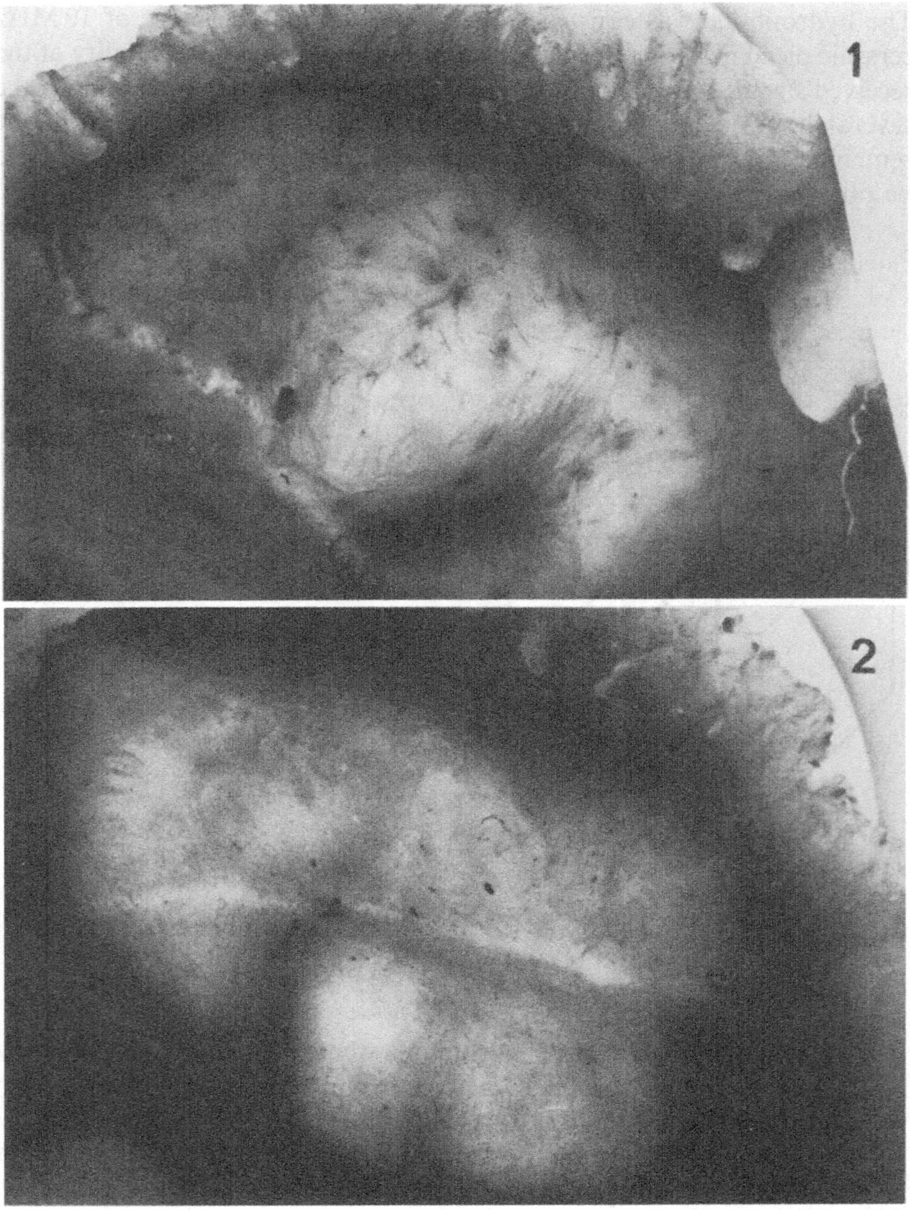

Fig. 2. Translumination photographs of the skull samples used. Numbers refer to Sample no. of Table 1

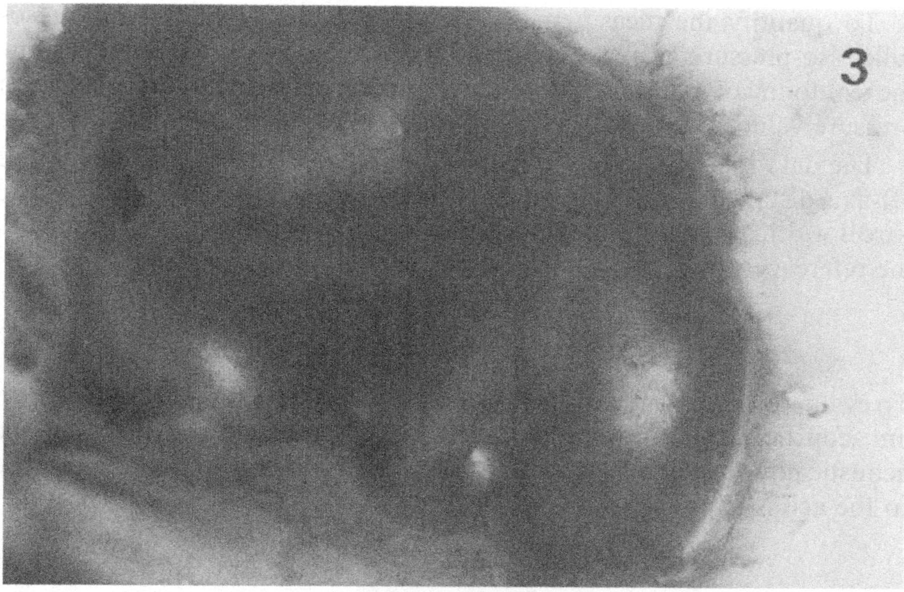

3

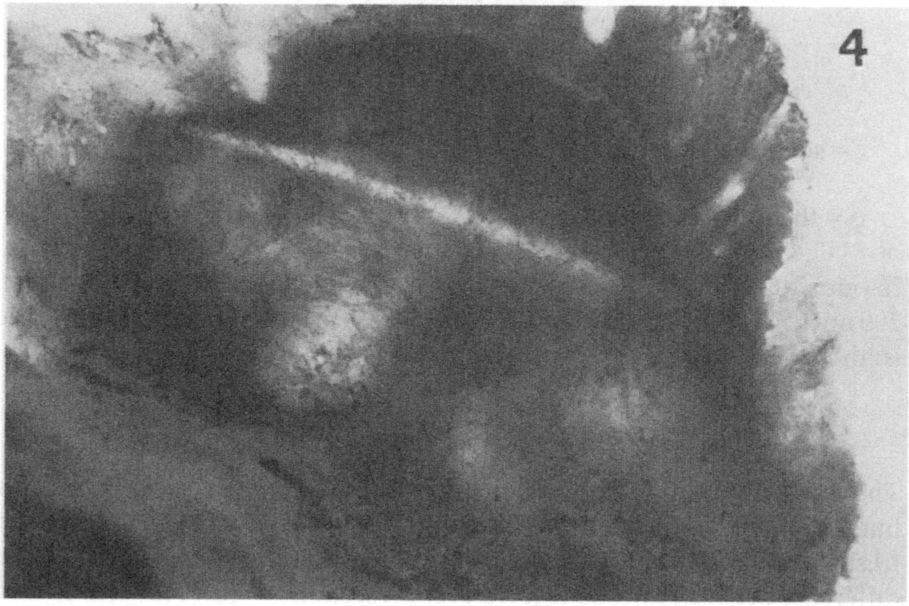

4

Next the x distance was increased by 1 mm and the same lateral scan was started. Eighty such scans were used to visualize the field in the x, y plane.

Scans in the y, z plane were made in the same manner from $y = 12$ mm and $z = -10$ mm with 1 mm steps in the positive z direction. To draw the data a special plotter program was used which showed the relative sound pressure as a function of the geometrical position.

To quantify the measurements, sound pressure contour plots or so-called iso-pressure graphs were made (Figs. 3 c and 4 c). These plots show the contours of constant pressure amplitude relative to the maximum pressure value in the focus (−3, −6, −12 dB).

The data in Table 1 were obtained from the iso-pressure plots and the off-axis distance was calculated from the y, z scans at x = 100 mm. For the −6 dB width at the x = 100 mm, the maximum at this distance was taken as the reference value.

Energy Measurements

To evaluate the transmitted energy and the energy loss, a microbalance with an acoustic absorber was used. With this equipment the time-average acoustic power was measured. Equation (1) relates the force on the balance to the acoustic power.

$$F = (2 * P_A * \cos^2(\varphi))/c \qquad (1)$$
$$P_A = c * F/(2 * \cos^2(\varphi))$$

P_A = average acoustic power (in Watts)

c = sound velocity in the solution used

φ = the angle of incidence (for absorbers this is 45 °)

In our situation $k/P_A = 68$ microg/mW where k is the force in microg. With 200 microg for the smallest measurable force, the minium detectable power is about 3 mW.

Skull Sections

There are several references in the literature to acoustic properties of the human skull. Some authors (White *et al.* 1967,1978) used formaline fixed or fresh samples. Fry and Barger (1978) showed that there was no significant difference between formaline fixed or fresh sections. White (1978) used fresh frozen samples stored in water after thawing. He did not observe any changes of acoustic properties over a period of months [2] .

For the experiments described here, dry samples were used. Before the experiment was started, the skull sample was put in water for several hours to eliminate the air inside of the bone.

The variations of the thickness of the investigated samples are shown in the photographs (Fig. 2). The thickness values in Table 1 are the arithmetical mean values of three measurements within the acoustic window.

Results

Field Without Skull

The ultrasound field was scanned for reference without a skull section. Fig. 3 a shows the relative sound pressure in the plane of the beam axis (x, y). The realtive distribution of the sound pressure in the z, y planes at

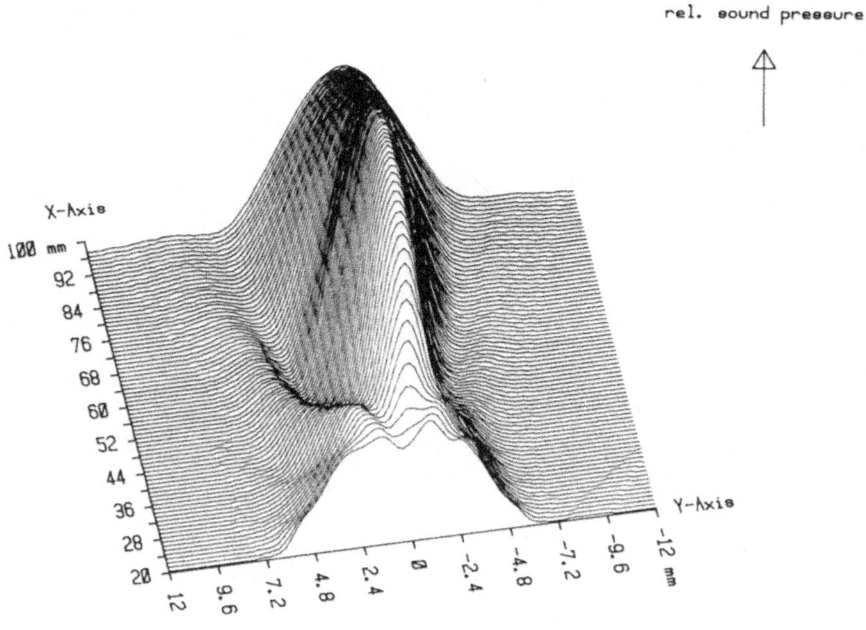

Fig. 3 a

Fig. 3. Transducer-field without skull sample. *a* Relative sound pressure in the x, y-plane for the field (z = 0)

x = 100 mm is plotted in Fig. 3 b. As expected, this plot had a rotation symmetry axis (x).

On the iso-pressure graph (Fig. 3 c), the maximum pressure was at a distance of 42 mm from the transducer surface. The beam width in the focus was 3.3 mm (−6 dB, Table 1). The axial −6 dB value was found at a distance of x = 97 mm and the −12 dB was outside of the measured region (x > 100 mm). In the right panel the maximum amplitude of every lateral scan was plotted relative to the absolute maximum. This depiction is like the silhouette of the relative pressure plot.

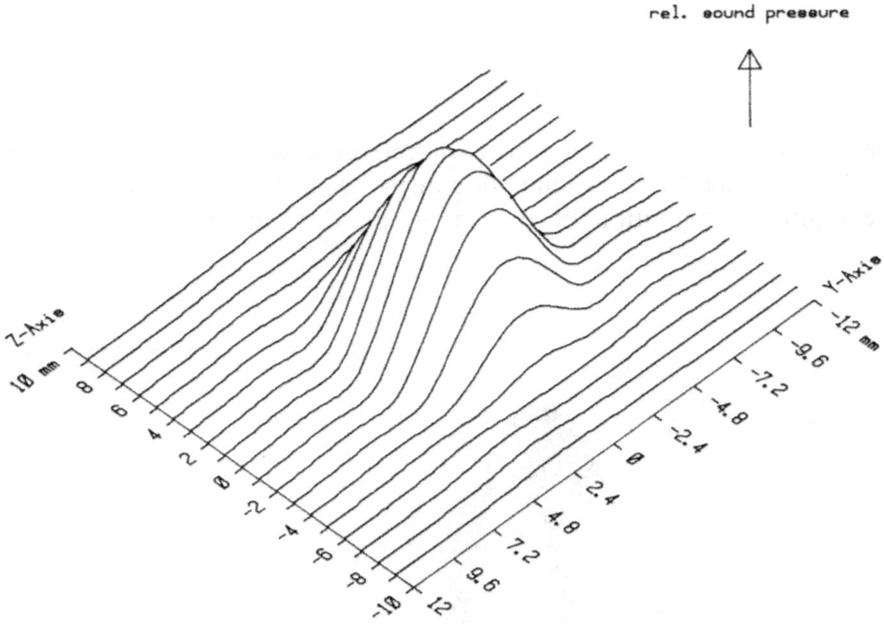

Fig. 3 b. Relative sound pressure in the z, y-plane x = 100 mm

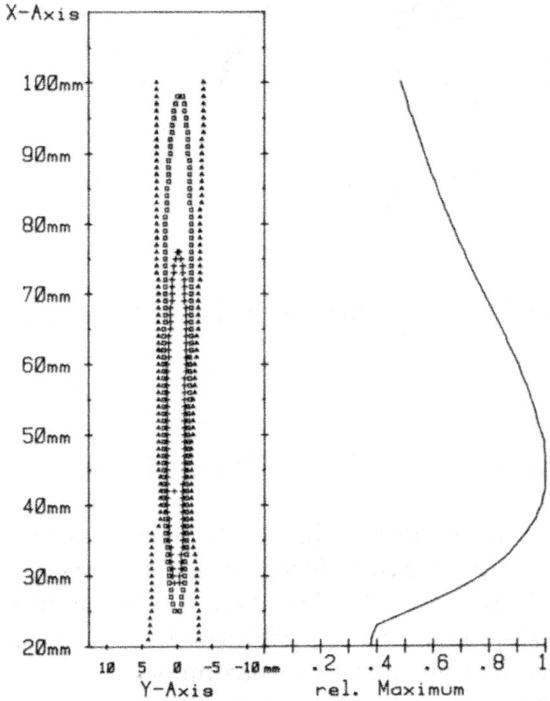

Fig. 3 c. Iso-pressure graph + = −3 dB, □ = −6 dB, △ = −12 dB, + = maximum

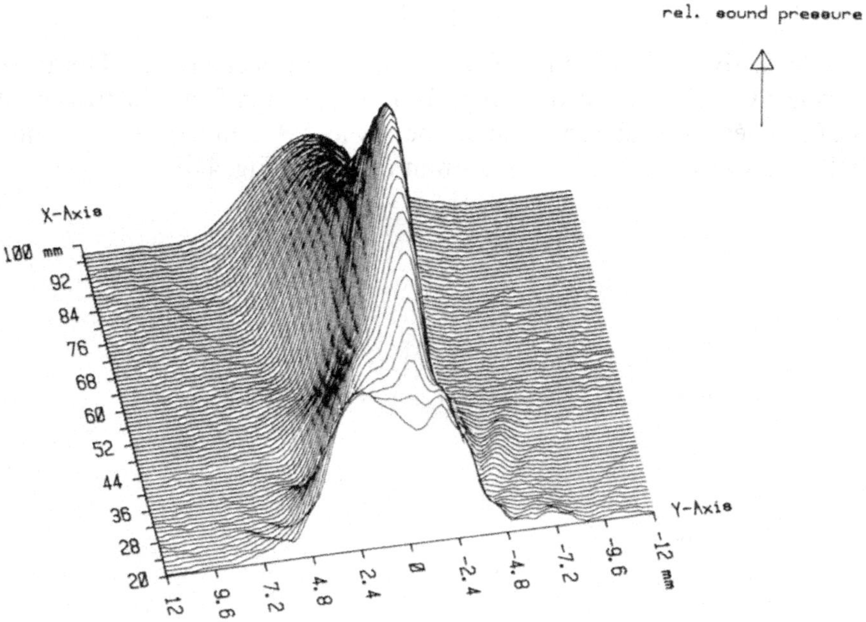

Fig. 4a

Fig. 4. Transducer-field with sample. *a* Relative sound pressure (x, y plane, z=0)

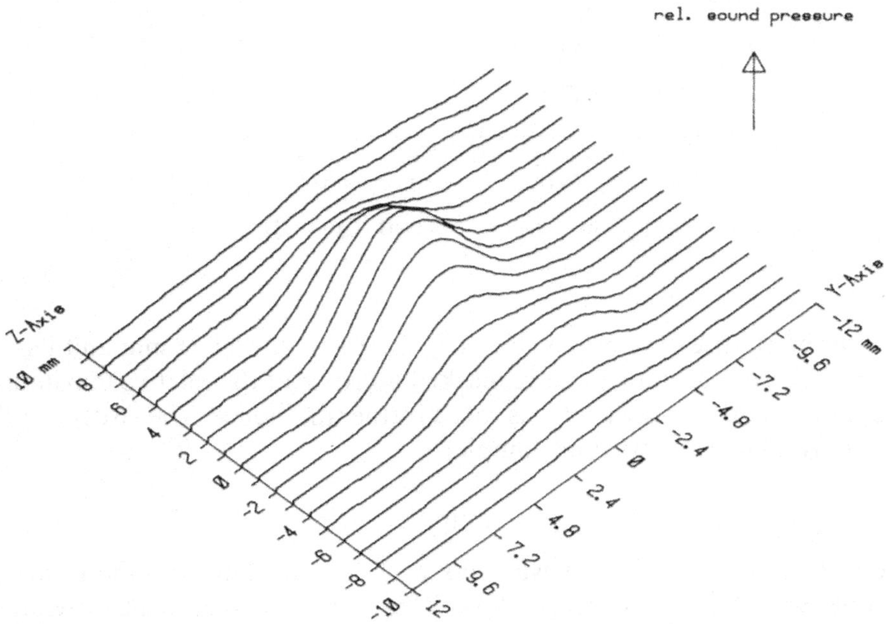

Fig. 4b. Relative sound pressure in x, y plane, x=60 mm

Fig. 4b. Relative sound pressure in x, y plane, x=60 mm

Sample 1

The skull was fixed about 1 cm in front of the transducer surface. The angle of incidence was close to zero degrees. In Fig. 4 no significant distortion of the beam is seen. A weak refraction in the +y and +z direction was found; the deflection at x = 100 mm was 1.6 mm (Table 1, Fig. 4 b).

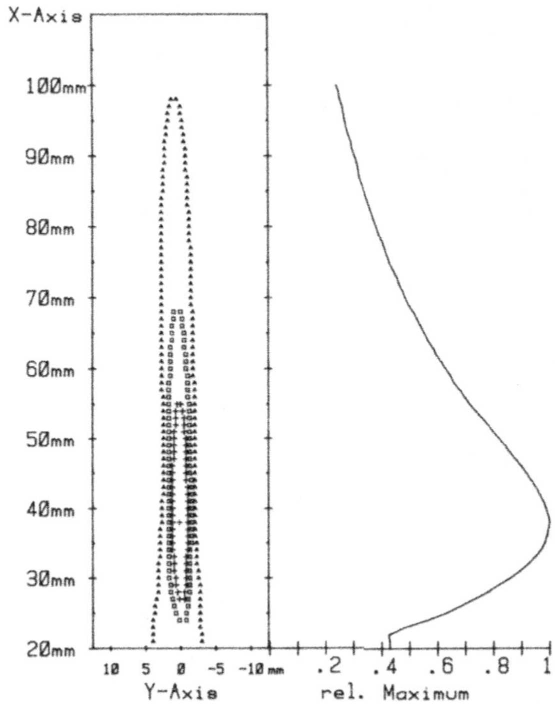

Fig. 4c. Iso-pressure graph + −3 dB, □ −6 dB, △ −12 dB

On the iso-pressure graph (Fig. 4c), the focus was at 38 mm and its — 6 dB width was 3.3 mm. A more marked decrease of the relative maximum amplitude on the transducer axis was a further difference. The –6 dB length was only 68 mm (97 without sample).

Sample 2

Here the angle of incidence was about 30 degrees. This was the thinnest sample with the lowest energy loss. There was no significant difference (except for energy loss) between this and the data without skull. The relative high angle of incidence induced no significant refraction (off-axis distance was 1.1 mm). The focal length was 46 mm and the −6 dB was 3 mm.

and the other with the main lobe. This is important for the resolution problems of an imaging system. Furthermore, the refraction limits the geometrical accuracy of such a system; mainly due to effects of variations of thickness. The broadening of the main lobe is a further limiting factor for the resolution.

Sample 3 with the nearest "focus" is also the sample with the highest energy loss. The narrowing of the maximum pressure distance (or focus) is not the lens effect but the effect of the scattered and refracted beam. It is difficult to estimate the reflected and absorbed part of energy. In other cases, however, the shorter focal length is the effect of the bone lens. The curvature of the bone forms a similar concavity to that of the lens. The resulting effect is that of using two focusing lenses. The second effect of the nearer focus is a shorter – 12 dB length. The consequence of this could be difficulties in obtaining good signals from deep arteries.

The present data suggest that it might be advantageous to use ultrasound lenses with a longer focal length. Then the focus behind the skull will be at longer distances so it is possible to improve the sensitivity of the Doppler instrument for vessels at a depth of 5–10 cm. Further experiments with other lenses will show if this is possible. The refraction as seen in some experiments cannot be corrected by a lens.

References

1. White DN Clark JM, White MN (1967) Studies in ultrasonic echoencephalography. General principles of recording information in ultrasonic B- and C-scanning and the effects of scatter reflection and refraction by cadaver skull. Med and Biol Engrng 5: 3–14.
2. White DN, Curry GR, Stevenson RJ (1978) The acoustic characteristics of the skull. Ultrasound Med Biol. 4: 225–252.
3. Fry FJ, Barger JE (1978) Acoustical properties of the human skull. Acoust Soc Am 63: 1576–1590

Author's address: P. Grolimund, Neurochirurgische Klinik, Inselspital, CH-3010 Bern, Switzerland.

3. The Doppler Principle Applied to Measurement of Blood Flow Velocity in Cerebral Arteries

R. Aaslid

The shift in frequency of a wave when either the transmitter or the receiver are moving with respect to the wave propagating medium was described by Doppler (1843). One of the earliest experiments to test this theoretical work was conducted by Buys Ballot (1845) with sound waves. In principle, sound and ultrasound are equivalent when deducting the formula of the frequency shift, whereas the deduction for electromagnetic waves will be different due to relativistic phenomena.

The Equation for the Doppler Frequency Shift

In a pulsed ultrasound Doppler instrument, the same transducer is used for both transmitting and receiving wave energy. The effect detected by this configuration is that of a frequency shift caused by a moving reflector. (For a description of the instrumentation see later section of this chapter.) The reflector—in our case the moving blood—has a velocity vector $\vec{v}$ which has an angle φ to the ultrasonic beam. The Doppler principle describes the effect of the component of the velocity vector along the line of observation. This velocity component or observed velocity, $\vec{v}$, is always lower than or equal to the magnitude $|\vec{v}|$ of the velocity vector.

The transmitted wave of frequency f_0 is propagated in the medium with a velocity c. The reflector moving with a velocity v will meet the wavefronts with a different frequency to that of stationary observers. This obvious effect has been felt by anybody trying to row or sail a boat against the waves in rough weather, an example which was employed by Doppler to explain the principle. If the velocity v is equal to c then the wave frequency perceived will be twice that of the stationary; if v is equal to $-c$ then the sailor will be riding with the waves and the frequency experienced will be 0. Thus there is simple linear relationship, Fig. 1, between the frequency f_1 encountered by the moving object and its velocity of motion along the propagation direction of the waves:

$$f_1 = f_0 (1 + v/c) \qquad (1)$$

The situation is slightly different in the case where waves of frequency f_1 are emitted by the moving object and received by a stationary observer.

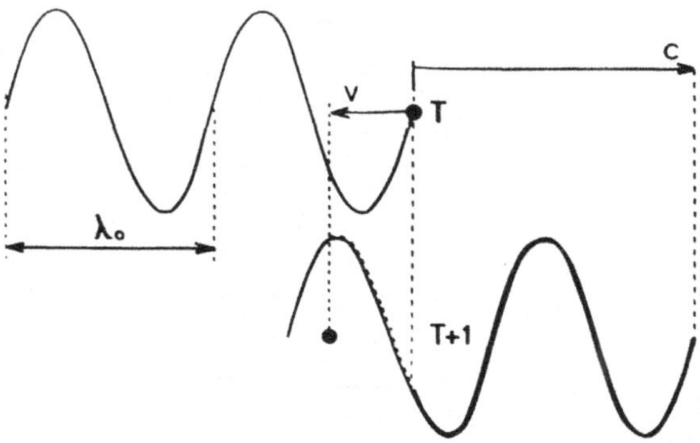

Fig. 1. Illustration of Doppler shift of a wave with wavelength $\lambda_0 = c/f_0$ when the receiver (filled circle) is moving at velocity v with respect to the propagation medium (and the stationary transmitter). After one time unit (T + 1), the position of the receiver and the wave will be as shown in the lower half of the figure. The wave has moved a distance c + v relative to the receiver, while it has moved only a distance c relative to the transmitter. Thus, during one unit of time, the moving object has received the additional part of the wave indicated by the solid + broken line in the figure. In this situation, the wavelength is constant, but the effective propagation velocity *relative to the receiver* is increased to c + v. The mathematical relationship for the wavelength can be formulated both with respect to the moving object and to the stationary transmitter, and these two expressions must be equal, therefore:

$$\lambda_0 = c/f_0 = (c + v)/f_1$$

Again the obvious example is the object moving at speed c: in the forward direction the wavefronts will pile up and the frequency perceived by a stationary receiver will approach infinity (supersonic bang). In the opposite direction ($v = -c$), the stationary frequency will be half of that transmitted because the wave is "stretched out" to twice length by the effect of the movement of the transmitter. As illustrated in Fig. 2, the wavelength λ_2 seen by the stationary observer will be related to the wavelength $\lambda_1 = c/f_1$ by the relation:

$$\lambda_2 = \lambda_1 (1 - v/c) = c (1 - v/c)/f_1 \qquad (2)$$

The received frequency f_2 is related to the wavelength λ_2 by the expression:

$$f_2 = c/\lambda_2 = f_1/(1 - v/c) \qquad (3)$$

Combining the two equations (1) and (3) the exact equation for the Doppler shifted received frequency is derived:

$$f_2 = f_0 (1 + v/c)/(1 - v/c) = f_0 (1 + 2 v/c + (v/c)^2)/(1 - (v/c)^2) \qquad (4)$$

This relationship applies all situations even when v approximates or is greater than c. For blood flow measurements $c = 1{,}540$ m/sec while $v < 6$ m/sec. The quadratic term will therefore always be smaller than 0.2%

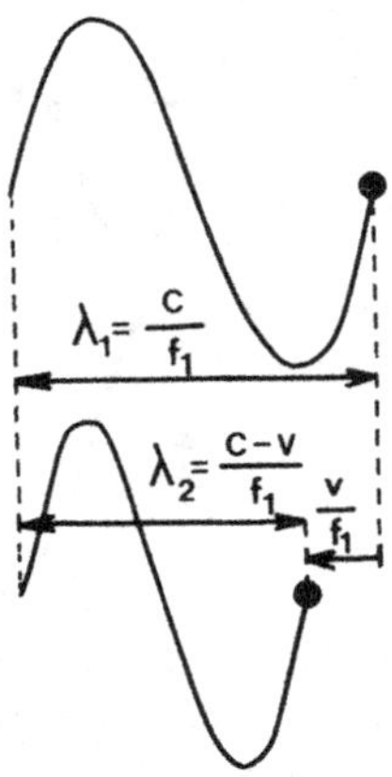

Fig. 2. Illustation of Doppler shift when the receiver is stationary and the transmitter (filled circle) of the wave with frequency f_1 is moving at velocity v with respect to the propagation medium. During the emission of one cycle, the transmitter moves a distance v/f_1, therefore the emitted wavelength must be this amount shorter than the wavelength of a stationary transmitter

of the linear term—for all practical purposes it can be neglected and we arrive at the familiar equation for the Doppler shift from flowing blood:

$$f = f_2 - f_0 = 2 \cdot f_0 \cdot v/c \qquad (5)$$

In this equation c can be considered a constant, thus for all practical applications the Doppler shift is proportional to the emitted frequency and the velocity. Although we have a free choice of f_0, practical considerations and equipment manufactures dictate us to use different frequencies for different applications. By rearranging the Doppler equation, the velocity component causing the frequency shift can be calculated:

$$v = 39\,f \qquad [2.0\,\text{MHz}] \qquad (6)$$
$$v = 52\,f \qquad [1.5\,\text{MHz}]$$
$$[v \text{ in cm/sec, } f \text{ in kHz}]$$

Expressing the Doppler shift in cm/sec (or m/sec) has the advantage that readings from instruments using different emission frequencies are immediately comparable. It may well be that future transcranial Doppler instruments will operate at different frequencies to optimize the signal to noise ratio. Indeed, recent experience in this laboratory indicates that an emission frequency of 1.5 MHz may be superior to 2 MHz in some applications because of better ultrasonic bone penetration. If readings are made in the cm/sec scale, no additional calculations are necessary to compare readings. Another very important advantage to this scale was

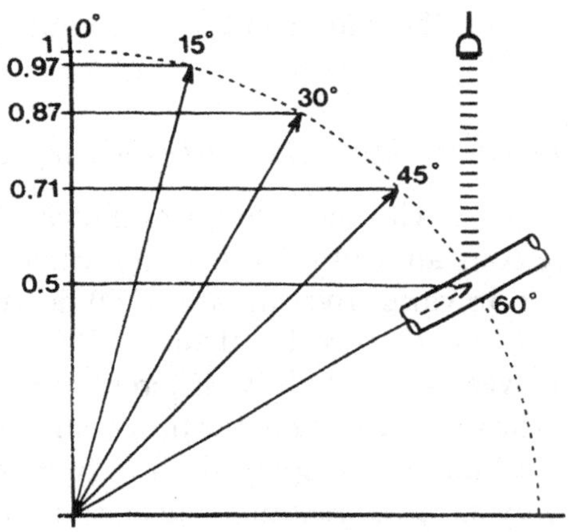

Fig. 3. Relationship between velocity vector (arrow) and observed velocity (component along vertical axis) for different values of the observation angle. For angles between zero and thirty degrees the observed velocity will be between 0.87 and 1.00 of the real flow velocity. For 60 degrees, only half of the real velocity is observed

stated by the Doppler Nomenclature Committee of the American Society of Echocardiography (1986):

"With regard to the Doppler content of the record, the committee recommends that the Doppler waveform should be calibrated in centimeters per second or in meters per second. We believe this to preferable to kilohertz calibrations since it provides a more physiologic means for communication of Doppler information as a velocity within the circulatory system."

While this statement was made for cardiac applications, the general intention is equally applicable to transcranial Doppler sonography.

Relationship Between Velocity Calculated from Doppler Shift and Real Flow Velocity

This disadvantage of the velocity scale is that it may allude to give more accuracy to the measurement than is warranted—an observer not sufficiently aware of the importance and implications of the geometrical relations might confuse absolute flow velocity with the velocity observed by the Doppler principle. This relationship between the two is indeed very simple, Fig. 3:

$$v = |\vec{v}| \cos\varphi \tag{7}$$

φ is the angle between the flow vector and the observation direction (the direction of the ultrasonic beam). In most recordings made with hand held continuous wave Doppler from peripheral arteries, this angle is unknown and calculation of flow velocity from Doppler-observed velocity would be very uncertain. However, there are some ways to improve the accuracy of the method:

Principle of Improving Accuracy by Insonating at Small Angles

The cosine function varies with the angle as graphically displayed in Fig. 3. We note the relative constancy of the function around zero degrees. When the angles of insonation varies over an arc of 60 degrees, from −30 to 30 degrees, the observed velocity is within 0 and −13% of the modulus length of the flow velocity vector. A slightly different view of this problem is displayed in Fig. 4: The relative error in the flow velocity estimate per degree error in the angle estimate is displayed as a function of the angle of insonation. While very accurate readings are possible at low angles in spite of considerable errors in the angle estimate, the errors will be significant at a 60 degree angle, and accurate readings are practically impossible between 70 and 90 degrees. These geometrical facts have their importance in duplex scanners for use in the carotid area: While these instruments allow compensation for the angle in the readings of velocity—some of the scan-heads are designed for insonation at blunt angles. Considering the function in Fig. 4, the accuracy would be greatly improved if the Duplex system could allow smaller angles of insonation. A method for using 2 MHz pulsed Doppler ultrasound for repeatable and accurate readings of absolute flow velocity in the extracranial internal carotid artery was reported previously (Aaslid *et al.* 1982), a more detailed description of this method can be found in the next chapter of this book.

For transcranial applications, we are anatomically restricted in the choice of insonation angle, since the availability of ultrasonic windows limits the approaches. Fortunately, even with these limitations of choice, the main basal cerebral arteries have an anatomy which facilitates accurate readings—at least when the main direction of the lumen is in the lateral-medial direction. These aspects are related to technique and are discussed in the next chapter. An indication of the technique independency of velocity readings is found in the published material on normal MCA, ACA and PCA velocity by different groups (Findings compiled in end of next chapter). The data are in close agreement, and testify that the strait-jacket imposed by the ultrasonic window may have at least one good effect—that of minimizing error caused by different operator techniques. (Another good effect is the rigidity of the cranium serving as a position reference when attempting scanning of the intracranial Doppler signals.)

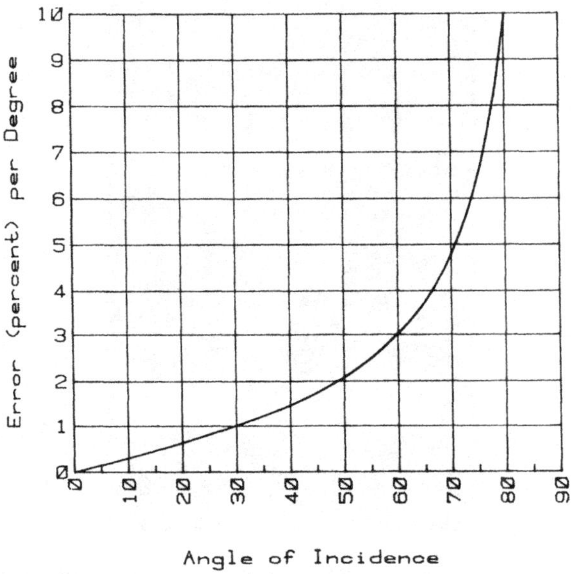

Fig. 4. Graph of the absolute flow velocity percentage error caused by a one degree error in estimate of incidence angle. The errors are very small for small angles, and increase steeply when the angle is higher than sixty degrees

Doppler Spectra and Their Relationship to Flow Distributions

The Doppler shift from blood flowing in arteries is not a single pure frequency such as that from a single moving reflector as described above. The signal received is a mixture of different frequency components coming from reflectors moving at different velocities. Examples of transcranial Doppler spectra are shown in Fig. 5. The spectral broadening effect is even more prominent in the transcranial approach than in cervical, peripheral or cardiac Doppler, because the sample volume size is relatively larger compared to the dimensions of the arteries. Thus, not only is the entire cross-sectional lumen insonated, but branches, different segments of curves and nearby vessels all contribute to the Doppler signal received. This consideration has two important consequences for the interpretation of transcranial Doppler signals:

1. The use of mean or mode frequency shift as indicative of spatial mean flow velocity is of dubious accuracy because we have no certainty of what the sample volume really encloses. Another fact against the use of mean frequency shift is the relatively poor signal to noise ratio found in transcranial signals. Therefore, the most practical Doppler reading of

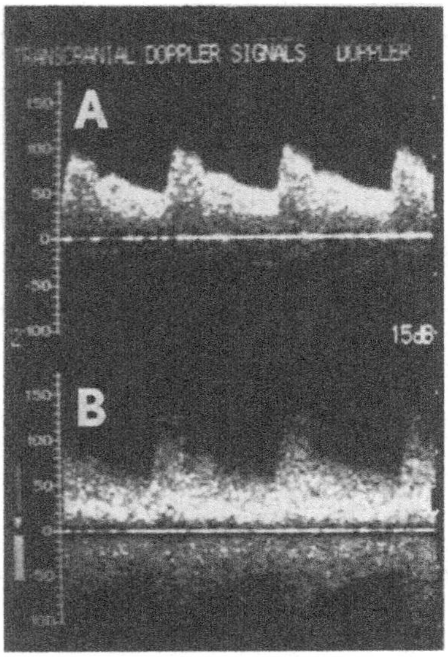

Fig. 5 A. Transcranial Doppler spectra from a straight segment of the MCA at a depth of 48 mm. A systolic window is seen, the main intensities of the spectra are concentrated within the upper half of the outline. The audible quality of this signal is "smooth" or "singing"

Fig. 5 B. Transcranial Doppler spectra from the region where the superclinoid ICA gives off the ACA branch. Signals from three vessels can be distinguished: the MCA and ACA as relatively weak positive and negative high velocity Doppler shifts while the ICA produces high intensity low frequency components above the zero-line. (The ICA is observed at a very blunt angle.) This sonogram its associated with an audible "gruffy" quality. However, this is a normal transcranial finding

velocity is that of the spectral envelope or outline. This parameter is relatively easy to define even if the signal level is barely above the instrument noise. Furthermore, if flow in curved segments is observed, the maximum Doppler shift will correspond to the part of the segment closest to being "in line" with the ultrasonic beam. The outline reading thus has an inherent error minimization when measuring absolute flow velocities.

2. Diagnostic criteria for disturbed flow such as the systolic window or spectral distribution which are used to assess low to moderate degrees of stenosis of the carotid bifurcation do not apply to transcranial readings.

These criteria are dependent for their accuracy on a relatively small sample volume, a situation which can only be met in very exceptional situations transcranially.

Bruit Spectra

An ultrasonic instrument designed to detect the Doppler effect will also be sensitive to phase and amplitude modulation of the reflected wave. These modulation modes create symmetrical sidebands around the carrier frequency, the frequency difference between the carrier and the sidebands being the same as the modulating frequency. An example of this can be seen if a vibrating tuning fork is held in front of the transcranial Doppler transducer (in air). The spectral analysis will show a prominent frequency at the fundamental of the tuning fork. In addition, higher harmonics of this fundamental wave will also be present if the amplitude of the oscillation is large. These higher frequencies are not necessarily present in the oscillatory movement of the fork, but may be created by the phase modulation process (Aaslid and Nornes 1984).

Phase and amplitude modulation of intracranial (and extracranial) ultrasonic echoes does occur if the beam is directed at a vibrating structure. In this mode, the instrumentation functions like a focused microphone, receiving phase modulated vibrations within the sample volume. The bruits detected together with the Doppler signals distally to a stenosis have been ascribed to this effect. Such bruits are also found in the intracranial circulation in a number of different types of pathology. They are probably caused by flow vortices impinging upon the vessel walls and setting up slight vibration of these and their surrounding structures. Sometimes musical murmurs are heard together with the Doppler signals (Aaslid and Nornes 1984, Harders and Gilsbach 1985) (p. 141). These phenomena are always associated with flow velocities above the normal range. The most likely explanation for the musical murmurs is the formation of a periodic vortex street, the flow being in a transitory state between silent laminar and full random turbulence.

Instrumentation for Transcranial Doppler Sonography*

Since the first reports of applications of the Doppler principle for measuring blood flow velocity (Satomura and Kaneko 1960, Franklin *et al.* 1961) there has been a considerable improvement in instrumentation. The addition of

* The instrumentation referred to throughout this book is the TC2-64 Transcranial Doppler manufactured by Eden Medizinische Elektronik GmbH (EME) of Ueberlingen, Federal Republic of Germany, or prototypes of this equipment constructed by the author and/or EME.

directionality resolution and the pulsed range-gated design (Baker *et al.* 1969, Perroneau 1969) as well as the combination with spectrum analysis and B-mode echo has made possible a sensitive instrument for obtaining data for analyzing the pulsatile hemodynamics of blood flow.

Measurement Principle

The principle of a pulsed Doppler instrument is illustrated in Fig. 6. Bursts of ultrasonic energy are transmitted at regular intervals with a burst- or pulse-repetition frequency (PRF). These bursts travel (at velocity c) toward

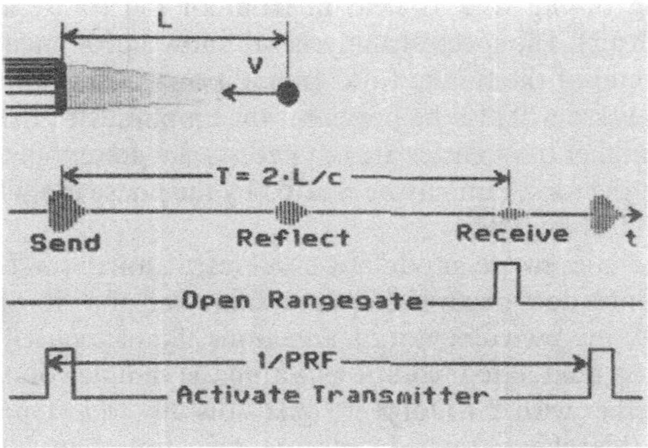

Fig. 6. Pulsed Doppler principle. *Upper* shows ultrasonic transducer emitting a beam at a reflector at distance L. *Middle* shows events with time as abscissa, and the two *lower* tracings represent internal signals in the instrument. See text for explanation

the reflector, the two being separated by a distance L. Some of the energy reflected travels back at the same propagation velocity. Thus, at a time $T = 2\,L/c$ after the emission of the burst, the reflected echoes come back to the transducer. The echoes are transformed into electrical signals and amplified. The principle of range-gating is in practice realized by an electronic gate which opens and samples the signal only for a short period around the time T. Signals arriving from reflectors at different distances arrive at different times and their effects are therefore eliminated from the sampled signal.

Range Resolution

In practice the range resolution is limited, the main reason being the bandwidth of the different components of the instrument and the length of the burst. For transcranial applications, the primary design consideration is a good signal to noise ratio. All other parts of the instrument being well-designed, this factor is determined by the noise bandwidth of the stages before sample and hold. This bandwidth can be reduced by filtering the received signal, but the side effect will be an increased length of the sample volume. This is one of the reasons that the instruments specifically developed for transcranial application have better signal to noise ratio, but

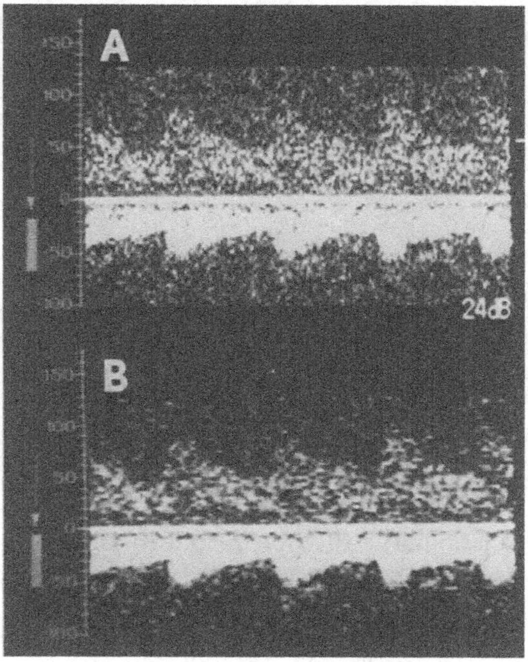

Fig. 7. Effect of signal averaging on appearance of spectrum: *A* shows a poor signal to noise Doppler signal without averaging. *B* shows exactly the same signal, but each spectral line is presented as a "sliding average" of 4 individual spectral lines. The background noise is greatly reduced

a larger and less defined sample volume than most other pulsed Doppler instruments.

Spectral Analysis

The Doppler shift is high-pass filtered to remove wall thumps and probe position movements, and the further information processing is usually fast Fourier analysis to display the spectral content of the Doppler signal. This mathematical procedure is performed digitally by a microprocessor in most modern equipment. The number of discrete spectral lines varies from 32 to 256 depending on the design. A 64-point transform will give better than 2% full scale resolution, this accuracy being sufficient for transcranial Doppler readings.

The intensity of a given spectral line is representend either by gray-scale, color or by "dot density modulation" (similar to gray-scale in printed reproductions). In transcranial Doppler applications with relatively poor signal to noise ratio, the best spectral representation can be achieved by using a closely spaced gray-scale with only 3 dB steps. This is equivalent to a factor of 1.41 between signal amplitudes = a factor of 2 in signal energy

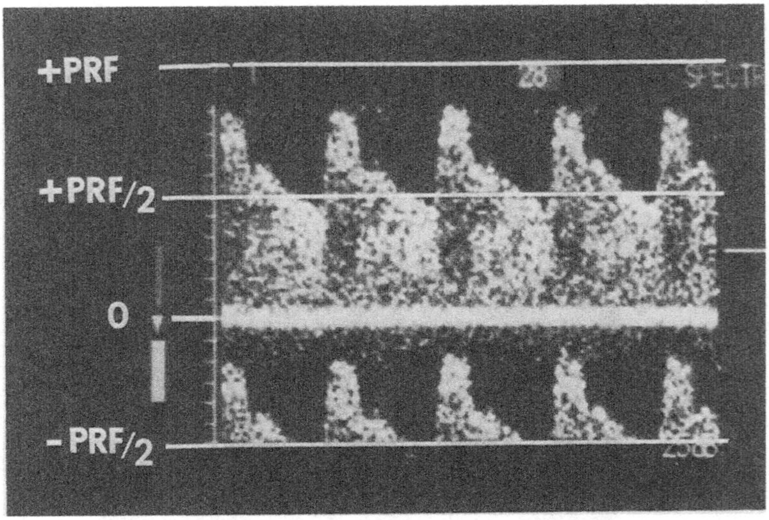

Fig. 8. Effect of aliasing: The PRF of the pulsed Doppler has been artificially lowered to 3 kHz to simulate under-sampling of the received arterial waveform with 100 cm/sec = 2.56 kHz systolic Doppler shift. Normally, only the signal between + PRF/2 and -PRF/2 would be shown, giving the characteristic aliased appearance. In the instrument used to produce this figure, the signals between 0 and -PRF/2 are also automatically added on top above + PRF/2 up to + PRF so that the observer will be in position to discriminate which of these representations is the correct one. In this case, there are no problems in recording a waveform with systolic Doppler shifts close to the PRF

difference = twice as many reflectors of ultrasonic signals going from one to the next higher level of gray.

With a low signal to noise ratio a better spectral display can usually be obtained by performing many FFTs and averaging these to reduce the random fluctuations of the spectral amplitudes. Fig. 7 illustrates the effects of this procedure: the lower panel shows the effect of averaging 4 of the transforms shown in the upper panel. The background noise is reduced, which is important when tracing the spectral outline.

Aliasing

The pulsed principle of the instrument has one important consequence: the information on the Doppler shift can only be sampled once during the pulse cycle. Doppler frequencies of f, f-PRF and f+PRF will in principle give the same values for all samples. This phenomenon is called aliasing (Nyquist theorem). If all Doppler shifts were known to be between -PRF/2 and PRF/2 this phenomenon would not give rise to problems in the spectral display. However, in transcranial Doppler recordings from spastic arteries or narrow collateral channels, Doppler shifts higher than PRF/2 are frequently observed. (The PRF is limited by the depth—in the conventional design, Fig. 6, the echoes have to return before the next burst is sent). Fig. 8 shows the effect in the spectral display of under-sampling of the received signals. The algorithm controlling the spectral display has been designed so that it shows frequencies between -PRF/2 and +PRF. Because of the aliasing, the band of frequencies (velocities) between -PRF/2 and 0 is the same as that between +PRF/2 and PRF. The systolic peaks give rise to Doppler shifts above PRF/2. and are thus reproduced both in the upper third of the display (correct) and in the lower third (unphysiologic). The observer understands this and there is no ambiguity in deciding which of these representations is correct. This ambiguity would arise when single spectral lines are observed. Fortunately the characteristics of physiological Doppler signals allow us to overcome this limitation of the pulsed principle.

Ultrasonic Transducer

The ultrasonic probe is a most important component of the instrument. The transducer is usually made out of a piezoelectric material that has a surprisingly high efficiency (80–90%) in converting electric to acoustic signals and vice versa. Normally, this piezoelectric disc would radiate equal amounts of energy in both directions. Letting the reverse side of the disc face against air prevents significant losses by this effect—and practically all the energy will be reflected and transmitted in the forward direction. As described by Grolimund in the preceding chapter, a plastic lens is used to focus the energy at a distance of 40 to 60 mm where the most important cerebral arteries are located. This focusing is effective both for transmitting and for receiving the energy. It is the focusing that makes it possible to record Doppler signals from narrow and small arteries (often less than 1 mm in diameter as in the ophthalmic artery and in spastic segments of the MCA) with a transducer that is 16 to 20 mm in diameter.

Transcranial Doppler Flow Mapping

A method for generating transcranial Doppler flow maps was reported in 1984 [1], two of the maps published are reproduced in Fig. 9. The upper panel shows the unretouched map with the sample volume placed at a depth of 59 mm where the ICA gives off the ACA branch. The lower panel shows a recording from the MCA at 50 mm with a superimposed drawing explaining

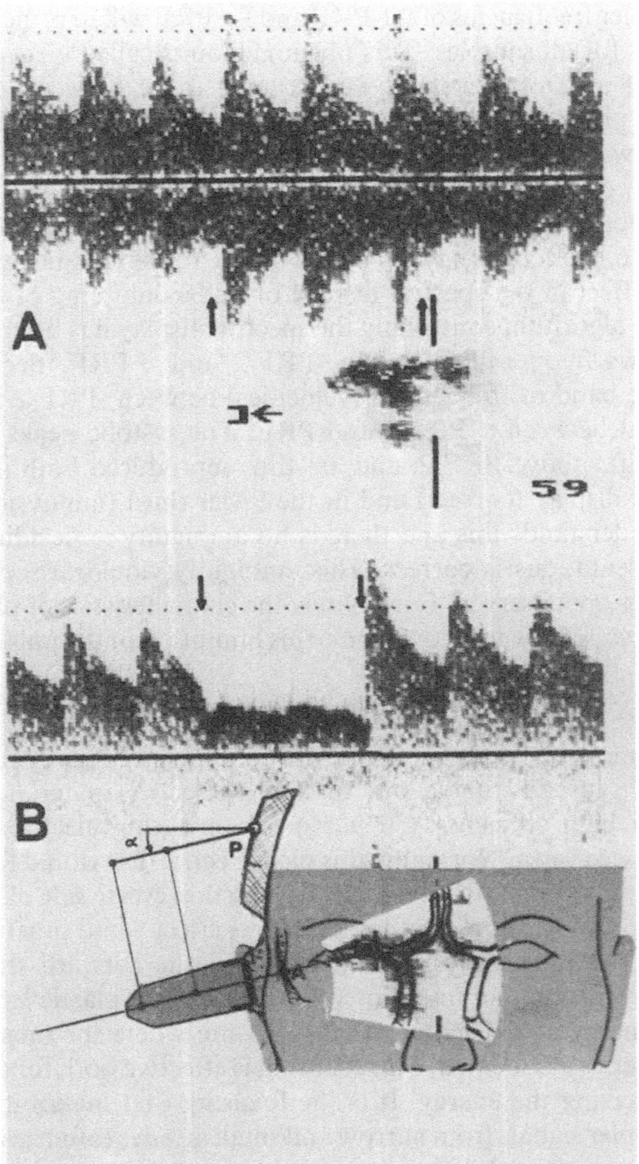

Fig. 9 A. Transcranial flow maps with spectra from terminal ICA, MCA and ACA. Test compression of collateral CCA is performed between arrows

Fig. 9 B. Schematics of mapping principle and recording of Doppler signal from MCA during ipsilateral CCA test compression (between arrows). See text for explanation of mapping principle. From: Aaslid R (1984) Transcutaneous evaluation of intracranial arterial flow. Proc Intern Conf, Application of Doppler ultrasound medicine, Duesseldorf

the mapping principle, and an explanatory outline of the arteries mapped. In this configuration, a sector of the coronal plane is displayed. A potentiometer mounted on a small platform, P, reads the tilt angle α. The other coordinate is the depth which was scanned to give a pseudo-multirange-gating effect. The platform was strapped on the head so that the ultrasonic beam would penetrate the cranium at approximately the same point A (ultrasonic window) independent of the tilt angle.

This arrangement could also be set up so that a sector of the horizontal plane was mapped. However, the two planes could not be mapped simultaneously. The dot density (=gray-scale) in the map describes the *intensity* of the Doppler signals. In subsequent clinical trials it became clear that although this system was useful in separating the signals from the anterior and posterior parts of the circle of Willis, it lacked the three-dimensional capability necessary to present the complex arterial network at the base of the brain.

A true three-dimensional display—although possible with present technology—would be very complex to generate, so that for practical purposes, two or three orthogonal projections are chosen to approximate space. The natural choice of projections are the horizontal, coronal (A–P) and sagittal (median) planes. In this book the two former projections are shown.

Multi-Projection Sample Volume Position Documentation

The relatively low degree of focusing that can be achieved in transcranial Doppler sonography does not encourage efforts in the direction of providing accurate anatomical flow maps, but a multi-projection diagram of sample volume position can be helpful in relating the different Doppler signals to their respective locations inside the cranial space. A detailed image is not necessary to achieve this end. Compared to the mental image guiding the investigator when performing a hand-held investigation, a projection display seen on the computer screen gives two distinct advantages: 1. it is more accurate and repeatable; and 2. it can be documented. Previously, Doppler imaging techniques were developed to aid diagnosis of plaques and stenoses of the carotid bifurcation (Spencer *et al.* 1974). However, this part of the circulation is less complicated and the need for a projection display to guide the investigator is felt even more imperative in transcranial Doppler sonography.

A new instrument has been developed on the basis on the initial experience with the two-dimensional configuration described above*. The

---

* Now manufactured by Eden Medizinische Elektronik GmbH (EME) of Ueberlingen, Federal Republic of Germany, as the "Trans-Scan" 3-dimensional transcranial Doppler scanner.

probe positioning readout is described in Fig. 10. It basically consists of two orthogonal angle readouts such as used for the first system. In addition, the probe position on the surface—or more precisely the position of the point 10 mm in front of the probe—is detected by potentiometers. This position

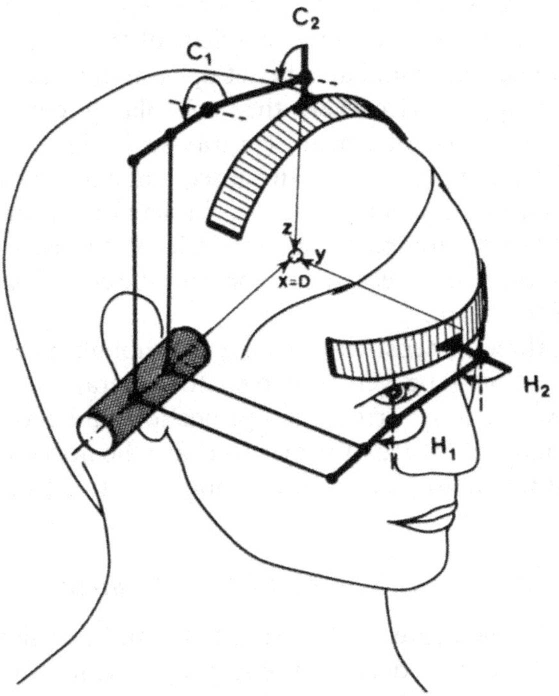

Fig. 10. Principle of two projection sample volume position documentation. The probe is connected by ball-joints and rods to scanning arms in the horizontal and the coronal planes. By computer readout of the angles C_1, C_2, H_1, H_2 and the depth D, the orthogonal x, y and z coordinates of the sample volume can be calculated. The scanning arms are fastened on curved pads that fit over the forehead and the dome of the cranium. These provide position references: the y coordinate is measured from the front of the forehead and the zero reference for the z coordinate is the top of the crown of the head. The origin for the x coordinate is the surface in the temporal region (when the probe is aiming normal to the sagittal plane, the x coordinate is equal to the depth, otherwise, x is a three-dimensional cosine function of the depth and two angles). Transcranial Doppler scans generated by this system are shown in Fig. 11

can be locked when performing a scan so that penetration through the same spot of the cranium can be achieved.

This system has the five degrees of freedom which are required for the transcranial examination. It is basically the responsibility of the operator to generate the display. For each sonogram recording, a dot is drawn by the computer in the two projections. The area of this dot is proportional to signal power. The color is blue (light gray) if the negative Doppler shift is stronger than the positive, or red (dark gray) if flow towards the probe predominates. The sample volume is represented by a circle together with a

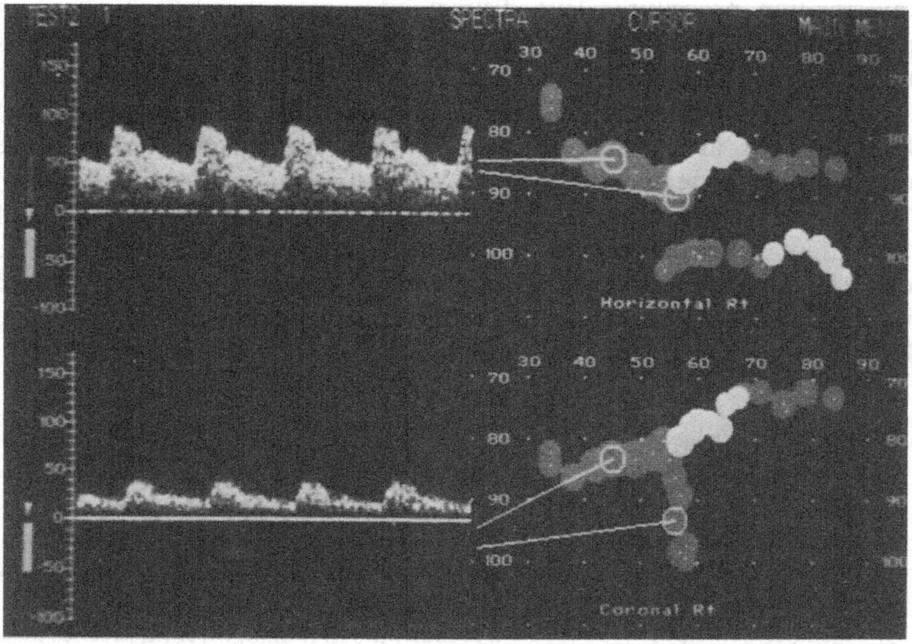

Fig. 11. Horizontal (upper) and coronal (lower) transcranial Doppler scans. The x coordinate is represented as the abscissa. In the horizontal display the y coordinate (Fig. 10) is the ordinate, in the coronal display, the z coordinate is the ordinate. The numbers of these coordinates represent millimeters, and a reference grid is indicated with a point at each centimeter. The two circles with white lines represent sample volume positions and beam directions for the two spectral recordings (MCA and ICA) shown in left panels. The dots representing recording points are dark gray (red) for flow predominantly toward the probe, and light gray (blue) for flow away. The circle of Willis is seen in the two projections. (For clarity the PCAs have been removed from the coronal display; they were found at exactly the same z coordinate as the ACAs)

line representing the direction of the ultrasonic beam. By recording multiple spectra from the various basal cerebral arteries, a composite display such as that shown in Fig. 11 may be built up. (The details are explained in the figure legend.) The spectra shown in the next chapter to explain the examination technique were recorded with this system.

As yet there is not sufficient experience to evaluate this approach, but the fact that a proper transcranial investigation depends very much on the skill of the operator to perceive and manipulate probe angle is a strong indication for using projection displays. In hand-held transcranial Doppler sonography, the depth is documented and used to differentiate between different signals. The described technique can be regarded as taking a further step along the path of more comprehensive documentation of the investigation procedure. Two distinct advantages have been noted in practical use: 1. The distance from the forehead to the circle of Willis seems to be relatively constant among adult individuals, which considerably speeds up the signal search procedure at the start of the investigation. This fact also helps artery identification. 2. When repeated measurements are made in the same individual, the system's permanent memory (disks) "remembers" the location of the ultrasonic windows and the positions of the different signals obtained. Then, because cranial landmarks can be defined with high accuracy, the follow-up procedures can utilize the stored information to shorten the examination time, and signals from the same locations and arteries can be compared.

References

1. Aaslid R (1984) Transcutaneous evaluation of intracranial arterial flow. Proceedings of Intern. Conference: Application of Doppler ultrasound in medicine, Duesseldorf, 1984
2. Aaslid R, Markwalder T-M, Nornes H (1982) Noninvasive transcranial Doppler ultrasound recording of flow velocity in basal cerebral arteries. J Neurosurg 57: 769–774
3. Aaslid R, Nornes H (1984) Musical murmurs in human cerebral arteries after subarachnoid hemorrhage. J Neurosurg 60: 32–36
4. Baker DW (1970) Pulsed ultrasonic Doppler blood-flow sensing. IEEE Trans Sonic Ultrason SU-17: 170–182
5. Doppler C (1843) Über das farbige Licht der Doppelsterne und einiger anderer Gestirne des Himmels. Abhandl Königl Böhm Ges Wiss, Ser 2: 465–482
6. The Doppler standards and nomenclature committee of the American Society of Echocardiography (1986) Recommendations for terminology and display for Doppler echocardiography. In: Kisslo J, Adams D, Mark DB (eds) Basic Doppler echocardiography. Churchill Livingstone, New York
7. Franklin D, Schegel W, Rushmer F (1961) Blood flow measured by Doppler frequency shift of back-scattered ultrasound. Science 134: 564–568
8. Peronneau P, Leger F, Hinglais J, Pellet M, Schwartz PY (1970) Vélocimètre sanguin par effet Doppler à émission ultrasonore pulsée. L'Onde Electr 50: 369–389
9. Spencer MP, Reid JM, Davis DL, Paulson PS (1974) Cervical carotid imaging with continuous-wave (CW) Doppler ultrasound. Stroke 5: 145–154
10. Satomura S, Kaneko Z (1960) Ultrasonic blood reograph. Digest, 3rd Int Conf Med Electron, London, p 254

Author's address: Dr. R. Aaslid, Institute of Applied Physiology and Medicine, 701 16th Avenue, Seattle, WA 98122, U.S.A.

4. Transcranial Doppler Examination Techniques

R. Aaslid

The first step in a transcranial Doppler examination is to localize a cranial "window" where the ultrasonic beam can penetrate without being excessively damped. It is necessary that the operator acquires the skill to optimize probe positioning and angle to achieve sufficient signal strength. The next step is that of identifying the signals from the different segments of the arterial network at the base of the skull. This identification is primarily based upon anatomical knowledge and sample volume position. The characteristics of Doppler signals from various segments and their response to compression maneuvers present further information for identification.

The subsequent sections summarize the present experience in examination techniques.

Ultrasonic Windows for Observing the Intracranial Circulation

Three main pathways to access the intracranial arteries have been described:

1. The transcranial approach to the basal cerebral arteries including the circle of Willis (Aaslid *et al.* 1982).
2. The transorbital route to the carotid siphon (Spencer 1983).
3. The suboccipital or transforamenal route to the basilar artery and the intracranial segments of the vertebral arteries.

A complete transcranial examination will usually incorporate all three approaches and it is thus possible to investigate a major part of the larger intracranial arteries. The transtemporal route is the main approach since it gives access to the ACAs, MCAs, PCAs and the carotid siphon as well as the collateral channels ACoA and PCoA.

1. The Temporal Window

The insonation from the temporal region has to be performed through solid bone tissue. This is only possible if the bones are thin (Chapter 2). In young adults it is usually possible to obtain good signals from a relatively large area, but in some elderly patients it may be barely possible to obtain signals through a very small window. Moving the probe just a few millimeters over the surface may cause a good signal to weaken and disappear. It is therefore important to move the probe slowly in small steps—always taking care to ensure good ultrasonic contact between the transducer and the skin. It is advantageous to rub ultrasonic gel into patients' hair and apply it to the skin surface in addition to the gel applied to the probe. Then, only moderate pressure is needed to maintain ultrasonic contact. Pressing too hard is inadvisable because it squeezes the gel away and may cause patient discomfort.

The temporal windows are found above the zygomatic arch. The approximate position of the arch can be palpated. Frequently, it is necessary to put the probe with its lower rim on the bulge over the zygomatic arch in order to direct the ultrasonic beam just over its superior edge. The windows are only rarely found more than about 3.0 cm superiorly to the zygomatic arch.

It is useful to discriminate between three different locations of the temporal window as shown in Fig. 1. The anterior temporal window (AW) is located posterior to the frontal process of the zygomatic bone. The posterior temporal window (PW) is found just anterior to the ear; in some cases this window is found more superiorly than the others. The middle temporal window (MW) is located between the anterior and the posterior temporal windows. Generally, the probe is aimed obliquely in a slightly posterior direction from the anterior temporal window; from the posterior temporal window it has to be aimed anteriorly to reach the arteries in the circle of Willis. The middle temporal window facilitates an approximately direct medial insonation.

In some cases all three temporal windows can be utilized for the examination, but the typical case presents only one useful temporal window. The posterior window is usually best in elderly patients. It is essential that all three areas are investigated to ensure the recordings are made from the best possible location.

Search for a Window

The search for the best window is complicated by the focusing of the ultrasonic beam and the relatively small dimensions of the basal cerebral arteries. Thus, it is not only necessary to locate an area in the cranium where the beam can penetrate, but also to aim the beam at a small target artery to obtain any Doppler signal. To minimize the latter problem, the search for the window can be performed with the depth setting of about 55 to 60 mm. At this distance, Doppler signals from the carotid siphon, the MCA, ACA and even the PCA are found, which increases the probability of obtaining signals.

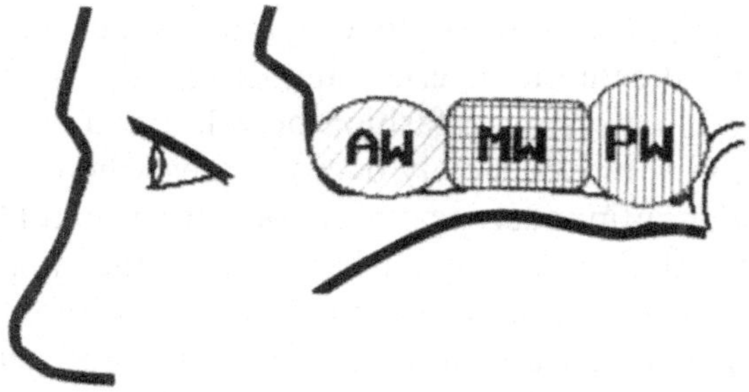

Fig. 1 A. Location of the temporal ultrasonic windows: *AW* anterior window. *MW* middle window, *PW* posterior window

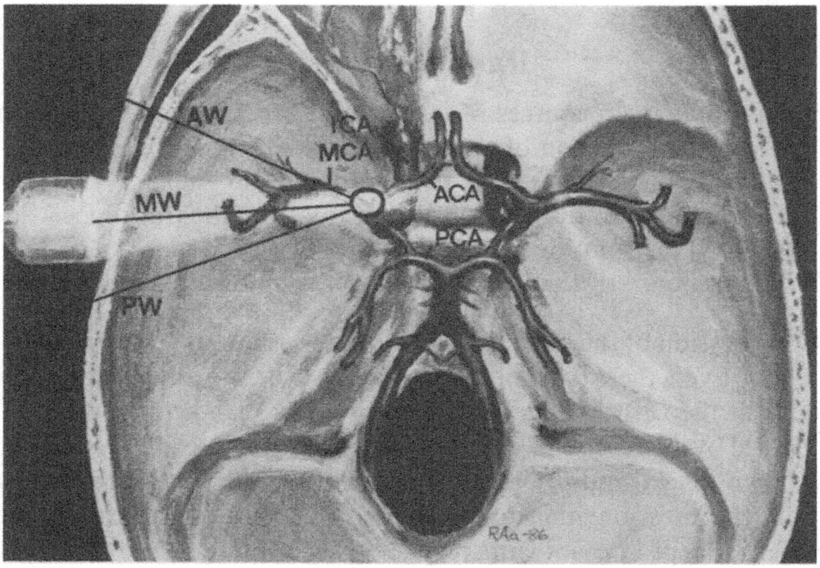

Fig. 1 B. Horizontal view of the circle of Willis and the insonation pathway through the temporal windows. The ellipse represent the sample volume. The arterial segments shown on this drawing represent approximately the territory that can be investigated by transcranial Doppler in a subject with good ultrasonic windows. *MCA* middle cerbral artery, *ACA* anterior cerebral artery, *PCA* posterior cerebral artery, *ICA* internal carotid artery. The posterior communicating arteries (PCoAs) are the narrow segments joining the PCA to the terminal ICA, the anterior communicating artery (ACoA) is the short segment joining both ACAs

During the search procedure, the investigator visualizes the approximate location of the basal cerebral arteries, and directs the probe accordingly. The probe is tilted in a scanning fashion both horizontally and vertically. The probe position is moved slowly over the area where the windows are likely to be found, continuously scanning for intracranial Doppler signals.

When an arterial Doppler signal has been found, it is important to proceed further and continually optimize probe position. The results of additional time spent in fine adjustment of probe with respect to the window can be rewarding in terms of signal strength and clarity of recordings. This type of "window optimizing maneuver" is required during various stages in the transcranial examination—when the probe position has been lost, when significant angle shifts are necessary to record from different arteries, and when the probe has had to be removed to apply more ultrasonic gel.

Artery Identification

There are three main sources of information for artery identification:

1. The spatial relation of the signal to other intracranial signals—this information includes both the depth and the angle of the probe.
2. The direction of flow (towards or away from the transducer) and the spectral distribution.
3. The response of the signal to compression or vibration maneuvers.

Compression of the common carotid artery should be performed low in the neck. Even then it involves a small risk of creating embolism from plaques in the carotid arteries. Therefore, this maneuver should only be performed by an experienced investigator after B-mode ultrasound imaging has shown the carotid arteries to be free of plaque. In the opinion of the author, compression maneuvers solely for artery identification are not necessary except in cases with very complex hemodynamic flow patterns. The compression maneuver can be, however, very valuable for determination of the capacity of the collateral network and this information may be essential in some cases.

Nonobstructive compression—or vibration—of the common carotid artery low in the neck is a less dramatic maneuver that can be employed to discriminate between flow coming from the ICA and flow coming from the vertebral arteries. However, considerable experience is necessary to evaluate and perform this maneuver.

By using proper examination techniques, it is generally possible to achieve a relatively high degree of accuracy in artery identification even without compression or vibration maneuvers. The main "landmark" for orientation is the branching of the superclinoid internal carotid artery (ICA) into the anterior cerebral artery (ACA). Using proper hand-held examination techniques, the operator can relate the spatial location of an unidentified signal to the landmark by "switching" back and forth between the unknown signal and the known.

Terminal Internal Carotid Artery (ICA)

After having found a suitable temporal window as described above, the termination of the ICA—defined as the location where it gives off the ACA branch—is identified by the following criteria:

ICA 1. With a depth setting of 55 to 65 mm, depending upon the diameter of the cranium , a Doppler signal is located. To avoid misidentification with siphon segments, the sample volume is scanned in the superior-inferior direction, since the signal from the most superior segments must originate from the approximate plane of the circle of Willis. The superior-inferior scanning routine is illustrated in Fig. 2. (A computerized system was used to generate this illustration, but the basic maneuvers will be the same in the hand-held techniques, with the operator creating a mental intracranial flow map). The Doppler shifts from the ICA may be considerably lower than those observed in the MCA/ACA due to the blunter angle of insonation. Exploration of sellar and cavernous components is usually possible by scanning even further inferiorly, where the Doppler shifts may be of varying direction and magnitude. Absolute determinations of ICA flow velocity are only possible from this window when the ICA has a predominantly lateral course.

It is also necessary to scan the sample volume in the anterior-posterior direction to clarify the relation between the anterior and posterior circulation. In most cases, the PCA is found from 1 to 2 cm behind the ICA in the plane of the circle (Fig. 6). Practicing these scanning or switching maneuvers is highly recommended. In the lack of a computerized scanning system such techniques are mandatory to achieve spatial orientation.

ICA 2. Flow in both directions is typically found at the flow divider at the end of the ICA (Fig. 2 A). It may be necessary finally to adjust the depth and probe angle to achieve this. The Doppler signals there typically have the "flow divider characteristics" with relatively strong components of low frequency shifts—the audible quality can be described as "noisy" or "gruffy". In some cases, the flow divider may be oriented in a different plane to the ultrasonic beam, then it can be difficult to display both directions simultaneously and very slight probe movements will be necessary to switch between ICA, ACA and MCA signals. Also, it is important to take into account that some cases with severe carotid lesions have reversed flow in the ACA.

ICA 3. The signal responds to ipsilateral vibration of the lower CCA. Compressing the CCA results in reversal of the ACA signal and diminish-

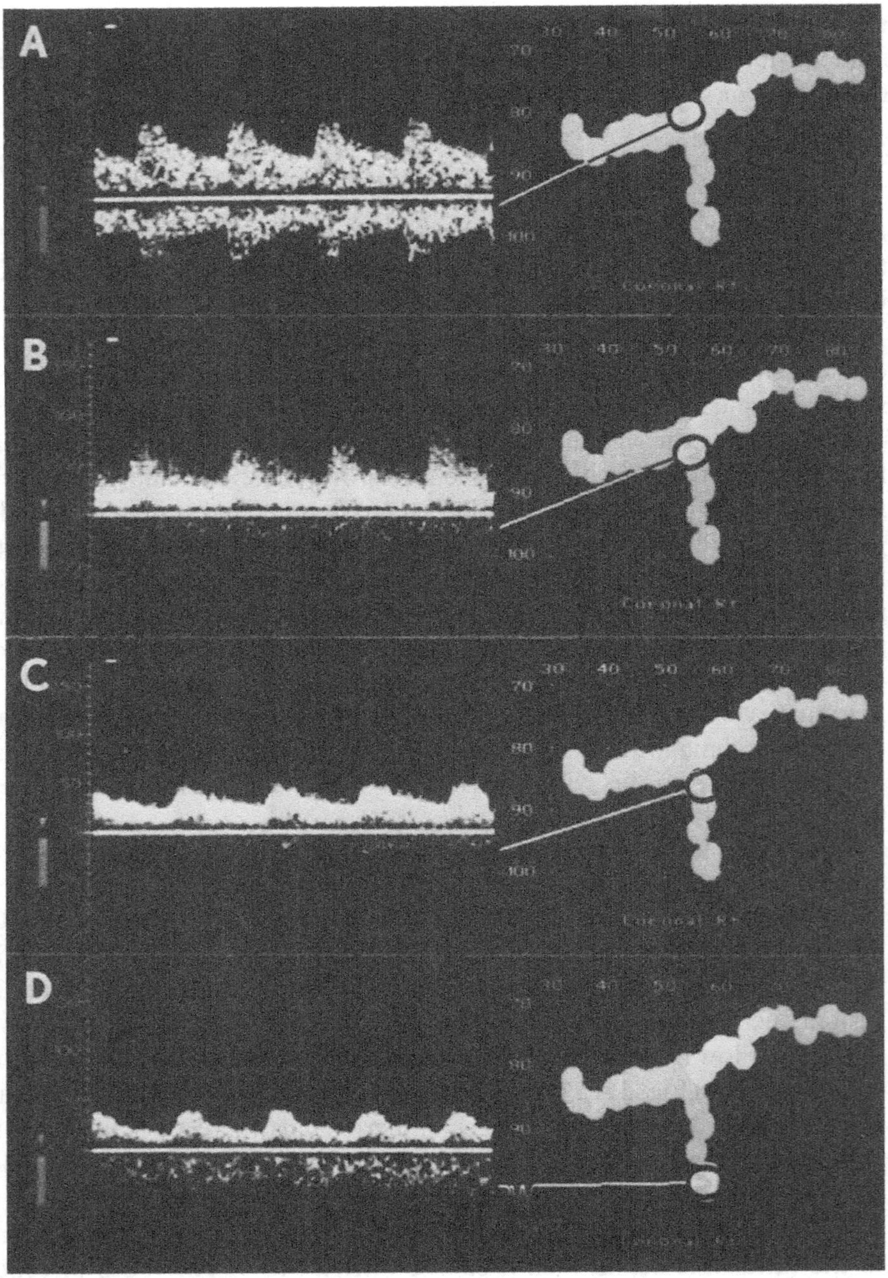

ment and damping of the MCA signal. If the sample volume is directed at the ICA below the ACA branch, compression usually results in complete cessation of flow.

Middle Cerebral Artery (MCA)

The MCA runs laterally and slightly anteriorly as a continuation of the intracranial ICA (Figs. 1 and 3). It has the highest volume flow of the branches from the Circle, carrying about 80% of the flow to the hemisphere (Toole 1984). An anterior temporal window allows almost zero degree insonation, whereas from a posterior window a somewhat blunter angle may be expected. The M 1 segment of the MCA, before its bifurcation (or trifurcation) allows estimation of the angle. While an accurate angle determination is not easy, it is also not necessary, because the essential information is whether or not the angle is sufficiently small to permit determination of absolute flow velocity. The relatively crude flow map obtained by transcranial Doppler techniques does provide this information. With the hand-held approach, the amount of angling necessary when scanning the MCA from 55 out to 35 mm gives the experienced investigator a feeling for the angle of insonation. Therefore, in this main cerebral artery, the Doppler readings will be sufficiently accurate to permit determination of flow velocity in absolute values.

The MCA is—together with its branches— normally the only artery seen between depths of 50 and 25 mm from the temporal window. The criteria for MCA identification are*.

MCA 1. The Doppler signal can be followed laterally with only slight probe movements from the termination of the ICA up to about 30 mm.

* *Note added in proof:* Recently it has been found that the middle meningeal artery can be confused with the MCA. Therefore, as described above (ICA 1) it is important to aim superiorly, and to explore the entire area where the MCA may be found.

Fig. 2 (Opposite). Investigation of the terminal internal carotid artery. *A* The sample volume is directed to the most superior position at the MCA-ACA branching point where both signals are observed. In this case the ACA velocities are slightly lower than those in the MCA. By directing the sample volume approximately 3 mm inferiorly, the signal changes character, *B* the MCA and the ACA components diminish (seen only as weak shadows in the figure) and the ICA components dominate. Three millimeters further inferiorly, only the ICA components of the spectra are seen, *C*. In this case the Doppler shift is low because the vessel is insonated at blunt angles. *D* shows spectra from the ICA probably within the cavernous sinus. A relatively high velocity venous flow is seen below the zero-line. The venous flow is still pulsatile, but the pulsatility is low compared to the arterial signal

MCA 2. The flow is towards the transducer. As illustrated in Fig. 3 C, the Doppler sound in the proximal segment of the MCA is "smooth" with relatively higher intensities in the upper frequency region of the spectrum, whereas broader spectra and lower frequency shifts are found at depths of 40 to 25 mm where the flow divides in a trifurcation (or bifurcation) into the MCA branches.

MCA 3. The signal responds to ipsilateral vibration of the lower CCA. (In cases with ipsilateral ICA occlusion this test does not apply.) The response to CCA compression is varying degrees of diminishment, depending upon the capacities of the collateral channels.

The Anterior Cerebral Artery (ACA)

The ACA, Figs. 1 and 4, is the last branch of the intracranial ICA. It starts out running medially, then turns more anteriorly until it approaches the brain midline and the anterior communicating artery. The best insonation is typically from a posterior temporal window because of the anterior course of the ACA. Furthermore, recordings made from the segment close to the branching off from the ICA gives the best chance of obtaining readings approximating true flow velocity, because the distal part of the A 1 segment may display a coiled and variable anatomical course. When different flow velocities are found at different depths (Figs. 4 A and B), this probably reflects variations in insonation angle. It is more difficult to develop a "scanning feeling" for this artery because it is shorter than the MCA, and located at a greater depth. The scanning technique gives an approximate indication of the relationship of the anatomy of this artery to the beam direction.

The ACA may be more difficult to identify than the ICA/MCA because: 1. it is usually smaller, giving rise to weaker Doppler signals, 2. it can display a tortuous anatomical course, and 3. the ACA flow direction may be reversed in pathological cases. If a bidirectional spectrum is found at the terminal ICA, the flow running away from the transducer represents the

---

Fig. 3 (Opposite). Investigation of the middle cerebral artery (MCA). *A* shows the segment of the origin of the MCA where a trace of the ACA negative Doppler shifts is still visible. *B* and *C* (depth = 43 cm, both horizontal and coronal projections represented) show sonograms from the middle of the proximal MCA segment. The relatively "top-heavy" spectra indicate that most of the flow cross-section have velocities above half of the outline velocity. The reaction to common carotid compression, *B* is an instantaneous diminishment in velocity, and a more damped pulse waveform. Autoregulation accounts for the gradual rise in velocity (and flow) after the initial drop. *D* (depth = 35 mm) shows low Doppler shift spectra from a branch of the MCA

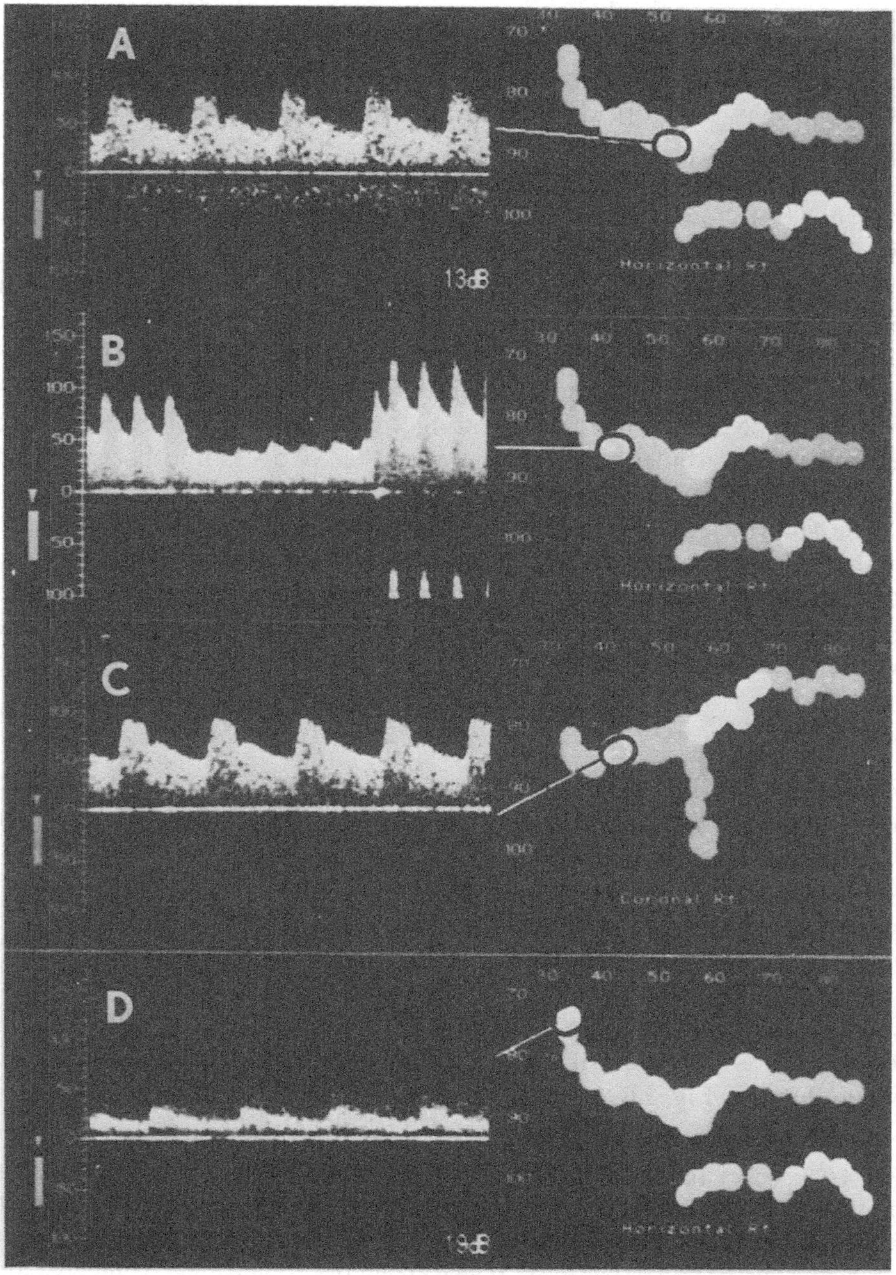
A
13dB
Horizontal Rt
B
Horizontal Rt
C
Coronal Rt
D
Horizontal Rt
19dB

proximal portion of the ACA. By scanning progressively deeper this signal can normally be followed down to the brain midline where it joins the contralateral ACA through the ACoA. However, in cases with tortuous ACAs, it may be difficult to scan the signal. The criteria for ACA identification are:

ACA 1. The ACA Doppler signal can be found at the ICA termination and it can be followed through increasing depths down to the brain midline, Fig. 4 A through C, Fig. 5 A.

ACA 2. The flow is away from the probe. In cases with occlusion or severe stenosis of the carotid arteries, the flow direction may be reversed due to its involvement in the collateral supply. This situation practically always leads to a significant increase in the flow velocity in the contralateral ACA which can be seen when investigating the other side. Moreover, high velocities and turbulence in the region of the ACoA is another sign that collateral flows are present, Fig. 5 B.

ACA 3. The response of the ACA signal to CCA compression depends on the collateral capacity of the anterior part of the circle of Willis. In most cases, the flow in the ACA reverses during compression (Fig. 4 C). However, the response is identical to that of the MCA (flow diminishment) if the ACoA is functionally absent.

The Anterior Communicating Artery (ACoA)

The anterior communicating artery is a small segment joining both ACAs in the brain midline, Fig. 1. Not much is known about the pattern of flow in this artery in normal physiology, and it is not seen in transcranial Doppler recordings unless its collateral function is provoked:

ACoA 1. The signal is found in vicinity of the region where both ACAs meet at a depth representing approximately the brain midline (70 to 80 mm).

ACoA 2. The flow is away from the side supplying the collateral flow, and characteristically there is a very localized area of very high velocities followed by a bruit type signal where the narrow ACoA jet empties into a wider channel, Fig. 5 B.

Fig. 4 (Opposite). Investigation of the anterior cerebral arteries (ACAs). *A* shows the most proximal segment (depth = 60 mm) where signals from the MCA are still quite strong, while *B* and *C* are taken at a depth of 66 mm where the ACA alone is represented in the signal. The lower velocity components in *B* and *C* compared to *A* could be due to the curvature of the vessel gradually increasing the insonation angle as depth increases. The ipsilateral CCA compression, *C* results in reversal of ACA flow direction, and autoregulation response similar to that in Fig. 3 B was observed. *D* (depth = 80 mm) shows signals from contralateral ACA. The same compression maneuver (Rt side) provokes high velocities in this channel due to its involvement in the collateral supply

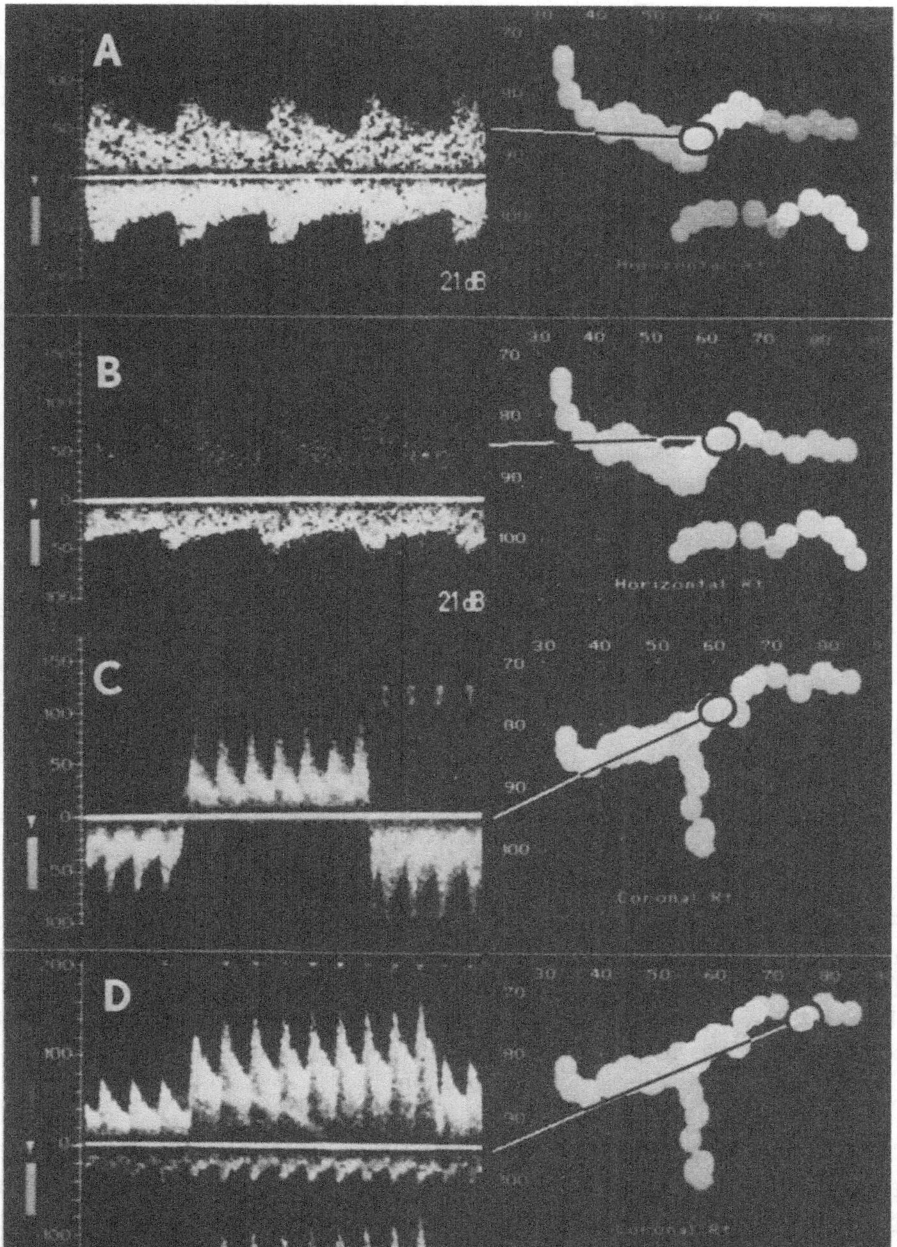
A
21dB
B
21dB
Horizontal Rt
C
Coronal Rt
D
Coronal Rt

The Posterior Cerebral Artery (PCA)

The PCA, Figs. 1 and 6, is most favorably insonated in the relatively short segment located close to the brain midline between the bifurcation of the basilar artery and the posterior communicating artery. This segment runs laterally before it curves more posteriorly and can be reached only with blunter angles of insonation.

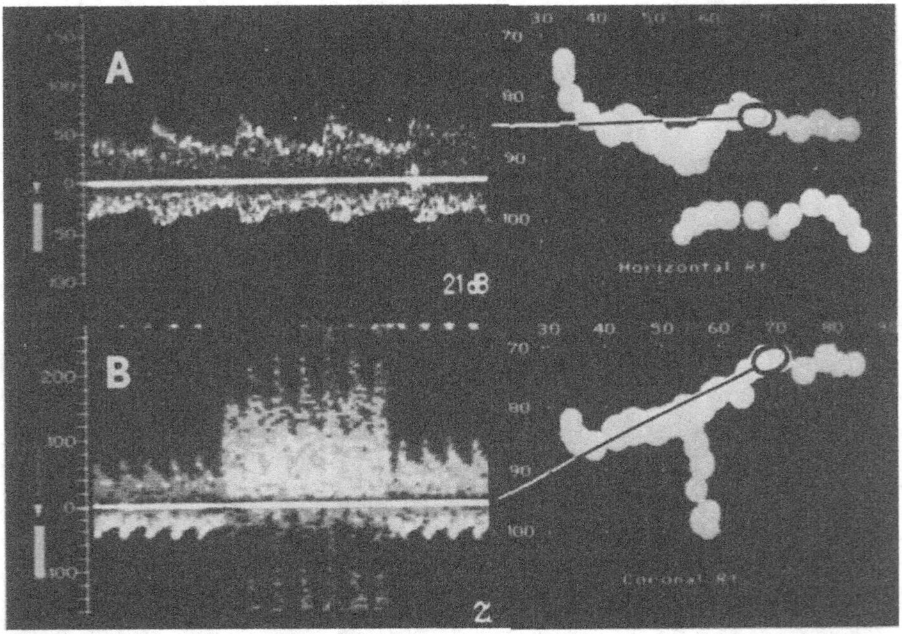

Fig. 5. Recording from the region of the anterior communicating artery (ACoA) at a depth of 72 mm. The display in *A* shows no sign of communicating artery flow. The two spectra represent both ACAs within the sample volume. However, when the right CCA is compressed, *B*, very high velocities and bruits are seen, since the collateral flow has to pass through the narrow communicating channel at this location

The search for the posterior cerebral artery is also started with the terminal ICA branching as a reference point, then setting the depth 5 mm deeper and directing the beam posteriorly. During this search it is often necessary to come back to the terminal ICA as a reference point to clarify the spatial relation of other signals received. The criteria for PCA identification are:

PCA 1. The signal found is located posterior to the ICA and the MCA and can be scanned down towards the brain midline. Moreover, the signal cannot be scanned further outward than about 55 mm, Fig. 6 A. This distinguishes it from the MCA which can be scanned up to 30 mm.

PCA 2. The signal from the most proximal segment of the PCA (closest to the midline) is towards the transducer, Fig. 6 B. The more distal segments may exhibit flow away from the transducer or even both directions simultaneously due to the curving of the vessel. Furthermore, at a depth corresponding to the brain midline, the signal exhibits "branching characteristics" with flow in both directions and a relative increase in the low frequency content of the spectra, Fig. 6 C. The Doppler shift of the PCA will always be lower than that in the MCA in the normal subject.

PCA 3. The PCA signal does not respond to a significant degree to vibration of the ipsilateral CCA. The effect of compression of the CCA is either augmentation, Fig. 6 B, indicating the participation of the posterior circle of Willis in collateral supply—or no change *.

In a relatively large percentage of the population, about 15%, the PCA stems directly from the ICA (in these cases the above criteria will not be applicable) and it becomes very difficult to identify these PCAs without a scanning system.

The Posterior Communicating Artery (PCoA)

Detection of absolute flow velocities in the posterior communicating arteries is very difficult due to the course of this artery which is almost perpendicular to the ultrasonic beam, Fig. 1. This artery is practically only observed when it is involved in collateral supply. The characteristics of the PCoAs are:

PCoA 1. The signal is found posteriorly and slightly inferiorly to the terminal ICA branching at depths approximately corresponding to the terminal ICA.

PCoA 2. The signals are provoked by ICA occlusion (or hemodynamically significant stenosis) and are seen as high velocities which may be in either or both directions depending of the orientation of the vessel with respect to the ultrasonic beam. Bruit type signals are then usually found at the location where the PCoA empties into the terminal ICA or the PCA.

2. The Orbital Window

It is recommended that the power output of the Doppler instrument is lowered for insonating through the orbital window to reduce ultrasonic exposure of the eye. However, no absolute levels for safe exposure have been established to date. Ultrasonic energies reported to produce cataracts in the lens are orders of magnitude above even the highest energies used for

---

* *Note added in proof:* Recently it has been found that the 10–20% change in PCA flow velocity when the subject opens and closes eyes can be used as a criterion of PCA identification to distinguish it from the superior cerebellar artery.

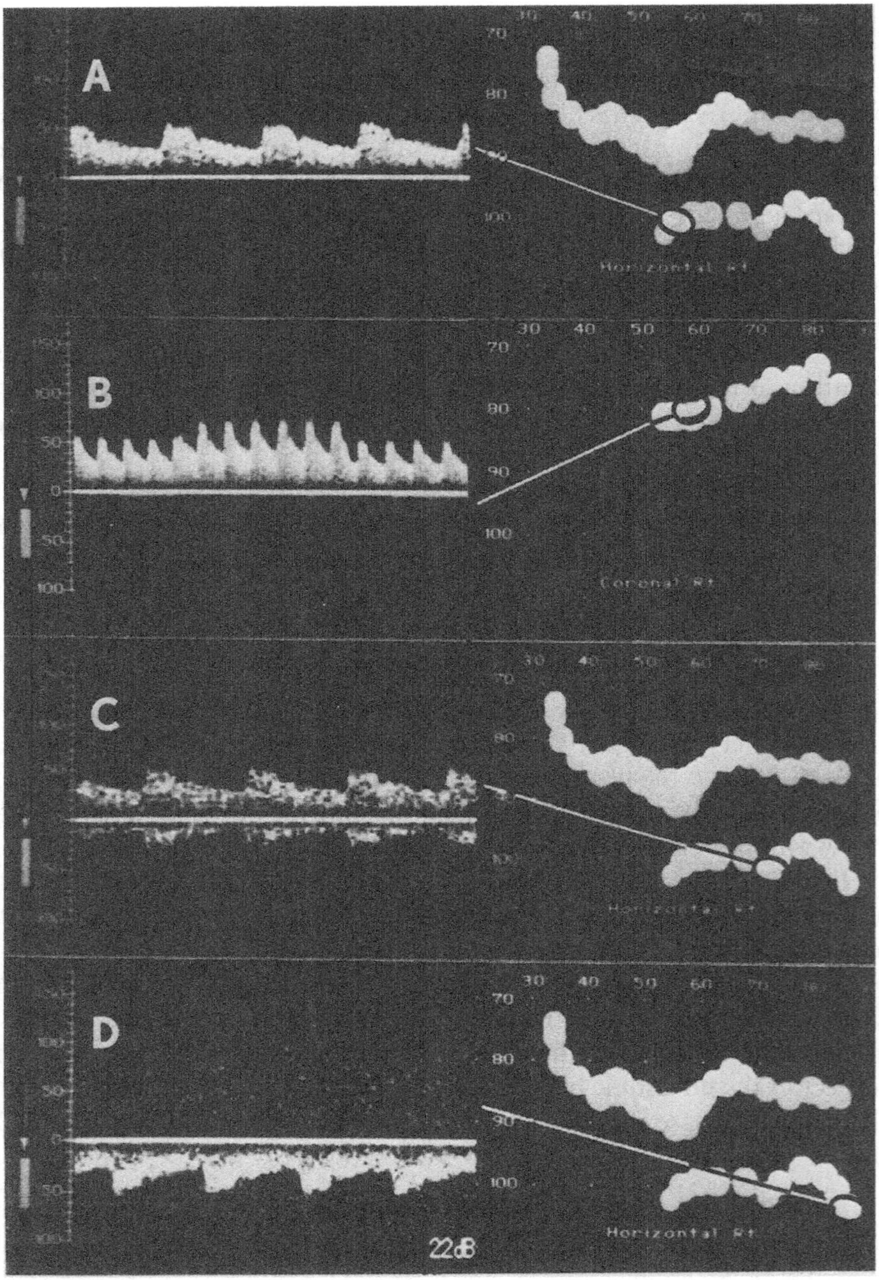

Fig. 6. Investigation of the posterior cerebral arteries (PCAs). *A* shows spectra (depth 57 mm) from the segment just before it curves posteriorly. In *B* (coronal projection shown) the sample volume depth has been moved to 62 mm, and the ipsilateral CCA has been compressed, resulting in augmented flow indicating the participation of this vessel in collateral supply. A recording from the basilar bifurcation is shown in *C* (depth = 72 mm). Signals from both ipsilateral and contralateral PCAs are seen. *D* (depth = 87 mm) shows spectra from the contralateral PCA

transcranial Doppler (Sokollu 1971). Contact lenses should be removed prior to examination. The transducer is placed over the closed eyelid with ample amounts of gel applied. It is then unnecessary to put pressure on the probe to maintain good ultrasonic contact. The ultrasonic beam is directed toward the optic canal with the depth set between 60 to 70 mm. It may be necessary to explore different placements of the probe over the eye to find the best insonation: Fig. 7 illustrates the probe postion.

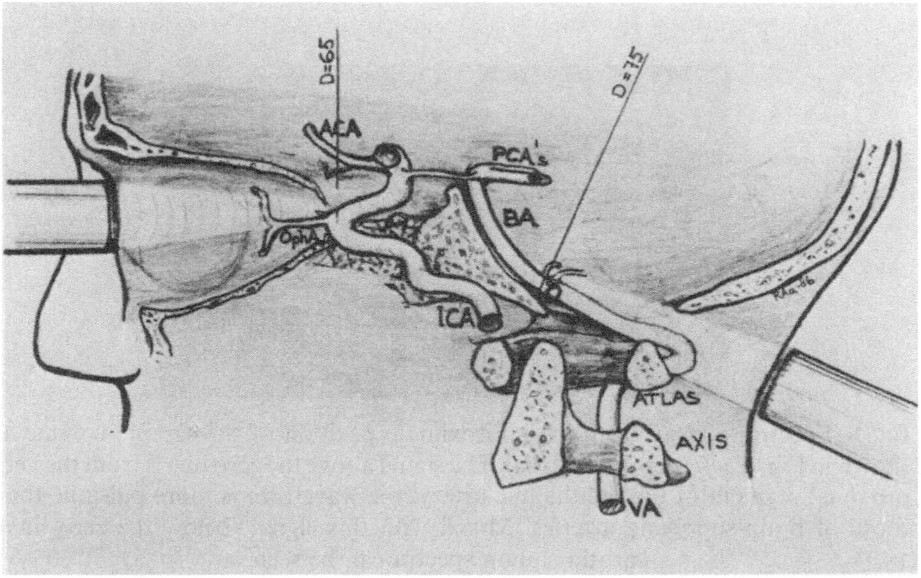

Fig. 7. Transorbital and transoccipital approaches to intracranial arteries. Parts of the carotid siphon can be insonated through fissures in the orbit and the ACAs can be observed through the thin orbital roof. The basilar artery and the intracranial portions of the vertebral arteries are insonated through the gap between the atlas and the occipital bone. *ACA* anterior cerebral artery, *ICA* internal carotid artery, *PCAs* posterior cerebral arteries, *BA* basilar artery, *VA* vertebral artery

The Doppler signals from the ophthalmic artery can serve as a reference point to the carotid siphon. The ophthalmic signals are towards the transducer, and have a characteristic pulse waveform typical of extracranial vessels, Fig. 8. They are found at depths from 40 to about 50 mm, at which distance none of the intracranial vessels are recorded. Progressively increasing the depth brings the siphon within range. The aiming of the probe should be mainly anterior-posterior with only a small tilt towards the median plane. Moreover the probe should be aimed in or slightly below the horizontal plane. At depths of 55 to 70 mm both the superclinoid, the genu and the parasellar components of the ICA can usually be insonated. Signals towards the probe are from the segments below the genu, while those indicating flow away are from the superclinoid region.

Recently it has been found that the ACAs can be investigated through an ultrasonic window in the orbital roof. This window is found by setting the depth at around 70 mm and directing the ultrasonic beam superiorly and medially from the position used to record from the siphon. To date the usefulness and possibilities of this approach have not been fully explored or documented.

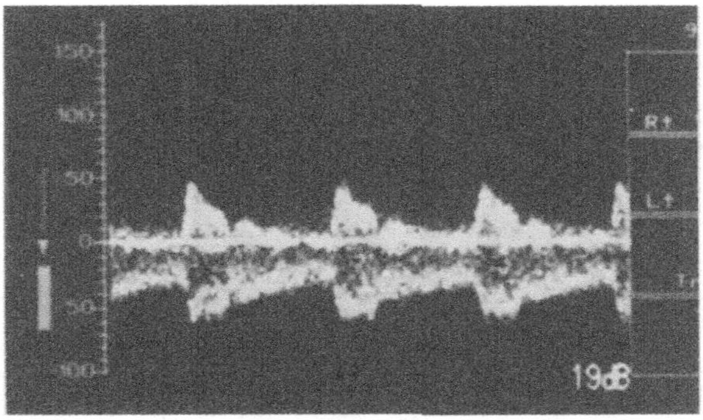

Fig. 8. Spectral display from the approximate position of the sample volume as shown in Fig. 7, *left* (depth = 65 mm). The signal above the zero line is from the very proximal segment of the ophthalmic artery, the waveform is more pulsatile than those of brain-supplying arteries. Mixed with this signal (below the zero line), carotid siphon spectra can be seen

The signals from the ACAs are mainly identified by probe direction, aiming more medially and superiorly than when insonating the carotid siphon. Identification of more specific segments of the ACAs is difficult without scanning techniques.

3. The Foramen Magnum Window

The vertical aperture size of this window is influenced by the posture of the patient and bowing the head forward with the chin down to the chest opens up the gap between the cranium and the atlas and facilitates the investigation. By insonating from the suboccipital region, Fig. 7, it is possible to explore the intracranial portions of the vertebral arteries and the proximal and middle segments of the basilar artery. In most cases, this insonation can be achieved by placing the transducer in the midline and directing the beam parallel to the sagittal plane. In some subjects the best results are obtained by a slightly oblique placement of the probe.

The basilar artery can almost invariably be insonated at angles smaller than 30 degrees, so determinations of absolute flow velocities are therefore possible.

The initial search for signals can be made with a depth setting of 60 to 70 mm. As with the other windows, the search has to include both changes in angle as well as probe positioning on the surface. The foramen magnum window is located at some depth, therefore some movements of the probe on the surface may be necessary to retain optimal signals when scanning the basilar artery down to 100 mm. Generally, the probe position has to be moved slightly inferiorly to obtain signals from the median and distal part of the basilar artery—if insonation is possible at all.

Identification of Basilar Artery

When a signal is found in the median plane at a depth of 85 to 100 mm and the direction is away from the probe, it can be identified as the basilar artery. The transition from vertebral to basilar artery flow is sometimes seen as a marked change in Doppler shifts going from depths of 90 down to 60 mm (depending on the size of the neck). When insonating the vertebral arteries the direction is perceived as lateral to the medial plane. Both these vessels can be investigated by moving the direction laterally from side to side. Signals from the posterior inferior cerebellar artery (PICA) can be seen at depths between 50 and 70 mm. The directionality of these Doppler shifts is typically toward the probe, in contrast to that from the vertebral and basilar arteries.

The Extracranial Carotid Arteries

Although the subject of this book is primarily the intracranial arteries, it should be mentioned that the extracranial channels are very easily accessible by the same instrument as used for the transcranial approach. A small adapter is cut at about 45 degrees from a silicone tube and mounted on the front of the transcranial probe as shown in Fig. 9. The space in front of the probe is filled with ultrasonic gel. In the experience of the author this gives a superior performance compared to smaller diameter 2 MHz probes because the beam can be better focussed with the larger transducer. The depth setting will be from 40 to 70 mm, depending upon the depth of the carotid arteries under the surface and how far distal to the bifurcation insonation is required. Beginning low in the neck, the common carotid artery is identified and the transducer arrangement is moved slowly in a cranial direction while listening for changes characteristic of the CCA bifurcation and the carotid bulb. Sometimes it may be necessary to increase the depth setting to scan further into the ICA and the ECA.

The enhanced sensitivity and penetration of the transcranial Doppler instrument permit detection of high velocities within even very narrow stenotic lumens. Moreover, the probe arrangement illustrated permits insonation of the ICA at angles lower than 45 degrees by slight tilting on the surface, thereby increasing the accuracy of the velocity determinations as shown in Fig. 4 of the previous chapter (p. 27).

In addition to its application in evaluation of carotid artery disease, the ICA flow velocity determination was found useful when monitoring

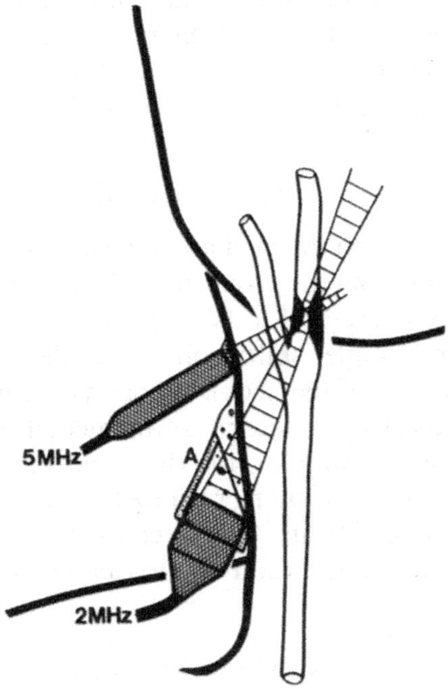

Fig. 9. "The shortest route is not necessarily the best." Method for using the 2 MHz transcranial probe for extracranial carotid examinations. An adapter A is cut from flexible silicone rubber tube. The 45 degree cutoff is filled with gel, and the probe is placed on the surface of the neck, allowing low angle insonation. For comparison of technique, insonation with conventional 5 MHz hand-held probe is also shown

patients with cerebral vasospasm. The day to day changes in ICA flow velocity were used as a reference value to evaluate whether changes in velocity in the MCA were due to lumen narrowing or caused by changes in brain flow (Aaslid *et al.* 1986).

Normal Values

Traditionally, systolic, diastolic and mean values are used to describe pressure, flow and velocity in the arterial system. Of these values, the mean carries the highest physiological significance because it depends less on central cardiovascular factors such as heart rate, contractility, total peripheral resistance and aortic compliance than do systolic or diastolic

Table 1. *Normal values of transcranial Doppler velocities reported in four different studies* (3–6)

		n	Mean ± SD	Systolic ± SD	Diastolic ± SD
MCA					
	(3)	50	62 ± 12		
	(6)	40	63 ± 9		
	(5)	50	65 ± 17	94 ± 23	46 ± 12
	(4)	30		94 ± 20	48 ± 10 (age < 40)
ACA					
	(3)	40	51 ± 12		
	(5)		50 ± 13	71 ± 18	34 ± 10
	(4)			72 ± 14	34 ± 7 (age < 40)
PCA					
	(3)	30	44 ± 11		
	(5)		40 ± 9	56 ± 12	27 ± 7
	(4)			60 ± 13	30 ± 7 (age < 40)
BA					
	(5)		39 ± 9	56 ± 13	27 ± 7
	(4)			64 ± 13	32 ± 6 (age < 40)

All values are cm/sec ± Standard Deviation. The frequency shifts reported in (4) and (5) were normalized by multiplying the kHz value with a constant factor of 39. No correction for insonation angle was attempted. Aaslid *et al.* (1982) [3], Arnolds and von Reutern (1986) [4], Harders and Gilsbach (1985) [5], Lindegaard *et al.* (1985) [6]

values. Moreover, the time-mean velocity correlates better with perfusion than the peak and trough values. If analysis of the waveform is of interest, the pulsatility index, as described in the next chapter, is a useful but relatively crude way of dealing with the problem. In the future, more exact methods such as Fourier waveform analysis will no doubt enter into clinical medicine because the instrumentation already includes a micro-or minicomputer that can perform these calculations without additional expense and time. The time mean value will not, however, become obsolete in this development, since it is indeed the zeroth Fourier coefficient. In view of this, when only one value is used to express the transcranial Doppler signal, it is recommended to use the mean and not the systolic or diastolic values.

Transcranial Doppler shifts from the various basal cerebral arteries in normal subjects were reported by Aaslid *et al.* [3], Arnolds and von Reutern [4], Lindegaard *et al.* [6], and Harders [5]. The results from these groups are summarized in Table 1. To facilitate the comparison, the formula: $v = 39f$ was used to convert between values of Doppler shifts expressed in cm/sec and kHz. The values reported are in close agreement, but in individual cases there is a considerable range of values of these Doppler shifts, with a relative standard deviation of about 90% higher than that reported for cerebral blood flow measured by indicator methods (Naratomi *et al.* 1979). Variations in insonation angle cannot account for this increased deviation, and the variability of flow velocity must therefore be attributed to differences of the cross-sectional lumen of the arteries. In addition to the absolute values as tabulated, some comments may be made on the values of relative velocities between different cerebral vessels:

1. The highest velocities are almost always found in the MCAs or the ACAs. More than 25% higher velocity in the ACA than in the MCA is an indication of an increased perfusion territory of the former. It should be noted that this could be caused by a variation of the circle of Willis where one ACA is hypoplastic. A hypoplastic ACA will usually not be evident from the transcranial investigation unless the signal to noise ratio is particulary good. One case reported by Aaslid *et al.* (1984) had 50% lower flow velocities in the hypoplastic ACA segment than in the contralateral ACA.

2. The PCAs and the basilar artery have lower Doppler shifts than the MCA in the normal subject. Therefore, the finding of relatively higher velocity in the posterior circulation is a strong indication of either increased flow in this part due to collateral effects or of arteriovenous malformations. When the increase is localized in a basilar artery segment it indicates arterial narrowing of this part. No report of PCA stenosis detected by transcranial Doppler has been found in the literature, but high velocities in spastic PCAs are seen after rupture of basilar artery aneurysms (unpublished observation).

3. The waveforms of the spectral envelopes as defined by pulsatility indices are practically identical in all cerebral arteries observed transcranially. Therefore, the finding of significantly lowered pulsatility in one or more of the cerebral arteries will raise the suspicion of some abnormality, the most likely being a stenosis of the supplying artery (see chapter on cerebral hemodynamics). Lowered pulsatility is also seen in AVM feeders. A significantly increased pulsatility has been observed in cases with large aneurysms. Increased intracranial pressure also results in more pulsatile waveforms, but the effect is then present in all cerebral vessels except in cases of extreme brain herniation. It should be noted that abnormal waveforms have also been seen in the PCoA and in the ACoA in rare types of circle of Willis variations.

The normal cerebral circulation presents transcranial Doppler signals free from vessel wall bruit caused by flow disturbances. Therefore, such phenomena do indicate either stenosis/spasm or volume flow above normal, caused by collateral effects, AVMs, hypercarbia or autoregulation breakdown. In younger subjects, a wall thump in early systole can sometimes be detected if the high pass filter of the Doppler instrument is below 200 Hz (8 cm/sec).

References

1. Aaslid R, Huber P, Nornes H (1984) Evaluation of cerebrovascular spasm with transcranial Doppler ultrasound. J Neurosurg 60: 37–41
2. Aaslid R, Huber P, Nornes H (1986) A transcranial Doppler method in the evaluation of cerebrovascular vasospasm. Neuroradiology 28: 11–16
3. Aaslid R, Markwalder T-M, Nornes H (1982) Noninvasive transcranial Doppler ultrasound recording of flow velocity in basal cerebral arteries. J Neurosurg 57: 769–774
4. Arnolds BJ, von Reutern G-M (1986) Transcranial Doppler sonography. Examination technique and normal reference values. Ultrasound Med Biol 12: 115–123
5. Harders A, Gilsbach J (1985) Transcranial Doppler sonography and its application in extracranial-intracranial bypass surgery. Neuro Res 7: 129–141
6. Lindegaard K-F, Bakke SJ, Grolimund P, Aaslid R, Huber P, Nornes H (1985) Assessment of intracranial hemodynamics in carotid artery disease by transcranial Doppler ultrasound. J Neurosurg 63: 890–898
7. Naratomi H, Meyer JS, Sakai F, Yamaguchi F, Shaw T (1979) Effects of advancing age on regional blood flow. Arch Neurol 36: 410–416
8. Sokollu A (1972) Destructive effect of ultrasound on ocular tissue. In: Reid JM, Sikov MR (eds) Interaction of ultrasound and biological tissues. US Department of Health Publication 73–8008
9. Spencer MP (1983) Intracranial carotid artery diagnosis with transorbital pulsed wave (PW) and continuous wave (CW) Doppler ultrasound. J Ultrasound in Med [Suppl] 2: 61
10. Toole JF (1984) Cerebrovascular disorders, 3rd edn. Raven Press, New York, p 9

Author's address: Dr. R. Aaslid, Institute of Applied Physiology and Medicine, 701 16th Avenue, Seattle, WA 98122, U.S.A.

5. Cerebral Hemodynamics

R. Aaslid and *K.-F. Lindegaard*

The principles of hemodynamics are the basis for understanding transcranial Doppler findings. Cerebral hemodynamics is a complicated subject because many factors are interacting. For example, the blood flow in a specific brain region is influenced by: 1. arterial pressure, 2. intercranial pressure, 3. hematocrit (viscosity), 4. degree of eventual proximal stenosis, 5. calibers and extent of collateral channels and 6. action of the cerebral autoregulation. It is the purpose of this chapter to describe the relationships between these factors and to serve as an introduction to hemodynamic interpretation of transcranial Doppler recordings in normal physiology as well as in patients with various forms of cerebrovascular pathology.

Cerbral Perfusion Pressure and Blood Flow

The energy for generating flow in cerebral arteries, capillaries and veins is provided by the left ventricle. The input, or gross driving force for the cerebral circulation is the pulsating pressure in the aortic arch as shown in Fig. 1. In this discussion all pressures are referred to a common hydrostatic reference point. (The center of the Circle of Willis could be defined as the reference point when transcranial Doppler recordings are involved. This Willisian point can be found accurately by transcranial Doppler scanning and it can be visualized with sufficient accuracy in hand-held techniques.)

The net driving force is usually defined as the perfusion pressure, which is normally the arterial blood pressure (ABP) minus the venous pressure (VBP). However, hemodynamics of veins is a much more complicated subject than that of the arteries. The pressure inside a vein can be equal to, or less than, the outside pressure. This causes collapse of the wall with the result that the flow resistance and inertia change dramatically. Consequently, central venous pressure is not an adequate parameter for use in defining CPP if the jugular veins are collapsed, which they normally are. Another possibility would be to define VSP (venous sinus pressure) as the VBP. The sinuses do not collapse even when the intracranial pressure (ICP) is raised above the sinus pressure (Nornes *et al.* 1975). However, the bridging veins connecting subdural veins to the sinuses do have soft walls. They therefore collapse and, as a consequence, the pressure in subdural veins does not fall below the intracranial pressure. At some point within a bridging vein there has to be zero transmural pressure as shown in Fig. 2. This means that venous pressure equals intracranial pressure. Distal to this point the flow enters a segment of collapsed vessel, within which the flow resistance cannot be defined by the normal vessel diameter. The flow resistance of collapsed vessels automatically adjusts itself (by varying the length and "tightness" of the collapsed segment) to match the pressure difference between the ICP

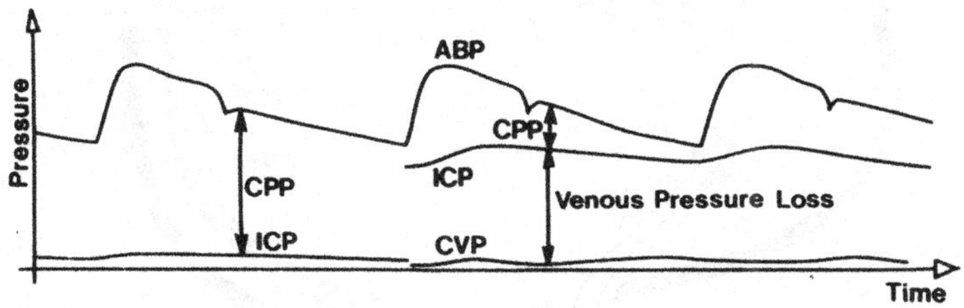

Fig. 1. Definition of cerebral perfusion pressure CPP. *ABP* is the blood pressure in the aorta. In the *left* half of tracings, the intracranial pressure (*ICP*) is normal. To the *right*, the ICP is elevated. Then the difference between ICP and central venous pressure (*CVP*) is causing venous collapse and increased outflow resistance, see Fig. 2

and the sinus pressure divided by the cerebral outflow. Thus, it is conceptually preferable to regard this part of the cerebrovascular resistance as being mainly governed by the intracranial pressure (sinus pressure being close to zero) and the CBF—rather than the conventional approach of assuming flow to be a variable of the resistance.

The term Starling resistance has been applied to this rather special pressure-flow relationship (Knowlton and Starling 1912). The flow in such collapsible tubes was analyzed by Fry *et al.* (1980). Because of this special property of the outflow from the subdural space, the convention has been chosen to define the cerebral venous pressure as equal to the intracranial pressure: VBP = ICP. The cerebral perfusion pressure (CPP) is then equal to:

$$\mathrm{CPP} = \mathrm{ABP} - \mathrm{ICP} \tag{1}$$

The definition of the cerebrovascular resistance (CVR) is as follows:

$$\mathrm{CVR} = \mathrm{CPP}/\mathrm{CBF} \tag{2}$$

or

$$\mathrm{CBF} = \mathrm{CPP}/\mathrm{CVR} \tag{3}$$

The (total) CVR can be visualized as a parallel connection of the different vascular perfusion territories of the brain. Within each territory the circulatory pathway consists of a serial connection of distributing arteries, arterioles, precapillary sphincters, capillaries, venules, and collect-

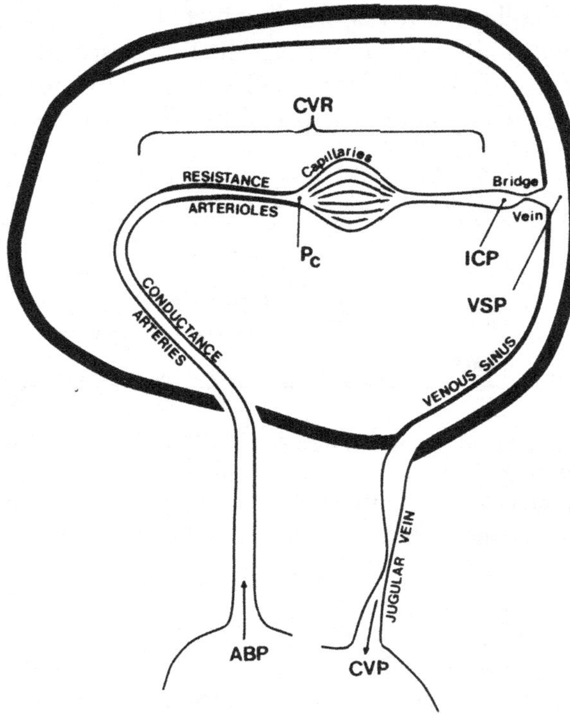

Fig. 2. Schematic diagram of the cerebral circulation. *ABP* arterial blood pressure; *Pc* precapillary pressure; *ICP* intracranial pressure (this is also the pressure within the bridging veins just proximal to the point where they collapse) *CVR* cerebrovascular resistance (mainly including small arteries, resistance vessels, capillaries and venules) *VSP* venous sinus pressure; *CVP* central venous pressure. Note that venous collapse can also occur in jugular veins

ing veins (Fig. 2). Much of the resistance within the cerebral circulation is found within the arterioles, including the precapillary sphincters. These segments of the serial connections can therefore be defined as resistance vessels. Micropuncture techniques have shown that there is a pressure drop from about 90 mm Hg in the distributing arteries (which normally contribute only minimally to the CVR) to less than 40 mm Hg in vessels of size 50 micrometers (Stromberg and Fox 1972, Kontos *et al.* 1978). The capillary pressure is about 20 to 30 mmHg. Obviously, the arterioles play a very important role in the total CVR—especially because they have the capability of regulating their calibers through vasomotor action of smooth muscle.

Cerebral Vascular Resistance: The Law of Poiseulle

The law governing resistance within a segment of a vessel was formulated by Poiseulle:

$$R = K \cdot \frac{8\mu l}{\pi r^4} \tag{4}$$

μ is the viscosity of blood, l is segment length, r is the vessel radius. K is a dimensionless constant which is always greater than, or equal to, one—the latter case representing the state of minimal loss flow with a parabolic velocity profile. In tubes of finite length, the energy loss will be higher because the optimal profile has not had time (space) to develop. Many of the distributing arteries in the human body fall into this category. The pressure loss will be particularly high in the first diameters of length of an inlet. These factors complicate the quantitative use of this equation on real flow situations in the circulation. Furthermore, the non-Newtonian property of blood (the viscosity μ is velocity-dependent) and the complex geometry make it even more difficult to calculate viscous resistance of a given part of the circulatory system.

There is one very important fact explained by the Poiseulle formula: flow resistance is inversely proportional to radius (or diameter) in the fourth power. A relatively modest decrease of 10% in vessel diameter results in a 34% increase in flow resistance. Halving the diameter increases the resistance by 16 times. Thus, the cerebral arterioles can produce a dramatic change in flow resistance by relatively small adjustments in caliber.

Carbon Dioxide Reactivity

The total cerebrovascular resistance is very sensitive to changes in arterial pCO_2. In contrast, the diameter of the basal cerebral vessels are only insignificantly responsive to pCO_2. Therefore, the flow velocity can be assumed to be proportional to CBF during CO_2 testing, and the transcranial Doppler can be used to study vascular reactivity of resistance vessels. Markwalder *et al.* (1984) found a CO_2 reactivity of $3.4 \pm 0.5\%$ change in V_{MCA} (velocity in MCA) per mm Hg change in end tidal pCO_2. This figure comes very close to data obtained in CBF studies, and confirms the assumption that the MCA diameters remains relatively constant during changes in pCO_2, the vasomotor action being confined to resistance arteries and arterioles. According to the Poiseulle formula (4), the 3–4 % change in flow resistance per mmHg of pCO_2 can be achieved by only about 1% change in caliber diameter of resistance vessels per mm Hg pCO_2.

This opens up the possibility of using the transcranial Doppler to test cerebrovascular reactivity in patients with cerebrovascular disease without having to use the complicated and expensive CBF methodology. Examples are shown in the chapters on AVMś (p. 99) and monitoring during cardiopulmonary bypass (p. 169). Bullock *et al.* (1985) found a significant decrease in reactivity in patients with severe carotid artery disease using rCBF methods, and this type of test should give similar results with the Doppler methodology.

Autoregulation of Cerebral Blood Flow

Assuming constant CVR, a change in perfusion pressure creates a proportional change in CBF. However, the tissue metabolic demands do not change. The brain possesses an intrinsic mechanism for adjusting the CVR to maintain constant CBF when the ABP is confined within reasonable limits (50 to 150 mm Hg). The autoregulatory mechanism is responsible for the puzzling observation that CBF is *not* reduced in moderate degrees of stenosis or spasm. The added resistance in the lesion is compensated for by peripheral vasodilatation lowering the resistance of the vascular bed so that the total resistance is constant.

The first effect to be considered is a reduction of cerebral perfusion as a result of an acute fall in CPP. Because the function of the central nervous system is dependent upon an adequate supply of oxygen, with vital functions failing after only a few seconds of hypoxia, there is obviously an imperative need of a fast acting mechanism to restore blood flow. The baroreceptor reflex of controlling arterial blood pressure acts to restore CPP, but the response is not very fast and it is sometimes ineffective. Acting in parallel to this, the intrinsic autoregulatory mechanism of the brain has a capacity for dilating resistance vessels (Fog 1937) thereby lowering the CVR to restore CBF. As shown in the subsequent section, this mechanism is very fast.

A second danger is associated with an increase in capillary pressure which is best understood with reference to Fig. 2. Assuming constant CVR, the pressure P_c at the entrance of capillaries will increase proportional to increases in CPP. There is a need to protect the thin membrane-like walls of the microvasculature from high transmural pressures. This can be achieved by fast acting vasoconstriction of proximal resistance vessels.

In addition to these protective functions, it is necessary to optimize cerebral perfusion to the metabolic need of the brain. Two hypotheses of the mechanism of cerebral autoregulation have to be considered, but which of these is ultimately responsible for the main autoregulatory action is still controversial (Strandgaard and Paulson 1984).

Myogenic Mechanism

The myogenic hypothesis (Bayliss effect) holds that an intrinsic property of the vascular smooth muscle of resistance arteries responds to changes in transmural pressure with parallel changes in muscle tone (Johnson 1980, Symon *et al.* 1973). It can be shown that this type of regulation distributed over a serial connection of segments can regulate a *pressure* somewhere within the arterioles (30 to 60 micrometers) when input pressure varies (Johnson 1980). The Bayliss mechanism should conceptually be considered as a pressure controller and not primarily as a flow regulator. However, regulation of flow would also result because the pressure at some point within the resistance vessels is kept constant. In most vascular beds of the organism, arterioles have been shown to respond in a manner which is compatible with this myogenic mechanism. Furthermore, isolated segments of cerebral arteries do react to increase in transmural pressure by vasoconstriction (Halpern and Osol 1985).

Metabolic Mechanism

The other hypothesis is that a feedback mechanism based on metabolic processes and vasoactive substances regulate flow. There is little doubt that the optimization and long-term regulation of CBF is based on this mechanism. Indeed, the strong reactivity of the CVR to changes in pCO_2 alone could explain at least some of the regulatory action. However, pCO_2 regulation cannot explain the fast response of the autoregulation because of the relatively high solubility of CO_2 in the brain. The size of the CO_2 compartment prevents rapid changes in concentration, thus slowing down the response to the time constant of this compartment. The relative slowness of such a metabolic mechanism led Symon *et al.* (1973) to postulate that the very rapid response observed in their experiments in apes was the product of a myogenic mechanism. Later findings (Winn *et al.* 1979) do not support this conclusion by showing that vasodilators such as adenosine could be the mediating substance. The concentration of adenosine has been shown to increase within seconds after cessation of brain circulation, and so there exists a possibility of a rapid metabolic feedback loop. However, it still remains to be shown conclusively that a mechanism based on metabolic products can explain the observed behavior of the autoregulatory response and to elucidate the relative contributions of the metabolic and the myogenic components of the cerebral autoregulation *.

---

* *Note added in proof*: In the section on autoregulation of cerebral blood flow it was stated that there exists the possibility of a rapid feedback loop through adenosine as a mediating substance. Since then, a series of experiments to determine the time-response of the metabolic component of the cerebral autoregulation have

Transcranial Doppler Observation of Cerebral Autoregulation

The relatively stiff walls of basal cerebral arteries have the consequence that the cross-sectional area of the flow changes minimally, even if CPP varies considerably. Indeed, if the compliance of these vessels is similar to that found in epicardial arteries (Reneman and Arts 1985), a 25 mm Hg change in arterial pressure would produce only a 2.5% change in vessel diameter. Therefore we may expect proportionality between flow and flow velocity, which opens up the possibility of using the Doppler velocity readings to measure changes in volume flow even when the perfusion pressure changes. When investigating relative changes in flow, preliminary comparison data (Fig. 7 in Chapter 11, p. 171) indicate that velocity V may be substituted for flow F. A study well under way confirms these findings for a larger series (Lindegaard *et al.*, to be published)

The dynamic response of the cerebral autoregulatory mechanism can be observed and analyzed from data obtained noninvasively in human subjects. Fig. 3 shows a recording made from the MCA of a 36 year-old female with an ABP of 120/85 mm Hg. In the time before the arrow, a lightly inflated cuff (<35 mm Hg) was held over the jugular veins on the low neck to increase intracranial pressure. The cuff was released at the arrow, causing an immediate rise of 33% in V_{MCA} which persisted over two to three beats. This rise was approximately proportional to the increase in perfusion pressure. After about 2.5 seconds, the regulatory response started to influence flow, and at 4 seconds, the V_{MCA} was already back to its pre-release value.

Almost exactly the same response was seen in recordings made during carotid surgery (Fig. 4) from a 70-year-old patient with very good collateral supply. The ICA clamp was introduced/released at the arrows (stump pressure was 30 mm Hg below the mean arterial pressure of 100 mm Hg). the autoregulatory compensation following unclamping was completed in less than 4 seconds.

---

been performed. (Aaslid R: Visually evoked blood flow changes in posterior cerebral artery. Manuscript in preparation.) As a response to alternating the stimulus to the visual cortex in an on/off manner (switching lights on and off), the flow in the PCA changed 15% in 10 normal subjects. The highest flow was observed eight seconds after the light stimulus was switched on, the half-time response was 2.9 seconds. The off response had a half-time of 4.7 seconds. Recording from the superior cerebellar artery (not involved in supplying visual cortex) no significant change in flow was observed. These findings indicate that the flow response to changes in brain function has a rapid dynamic action and support the view that the metabolic mechanism is responsible for both the fast response to blood pressure variations as well as the overall optimization and tuning of brain blood flow to metabolism.

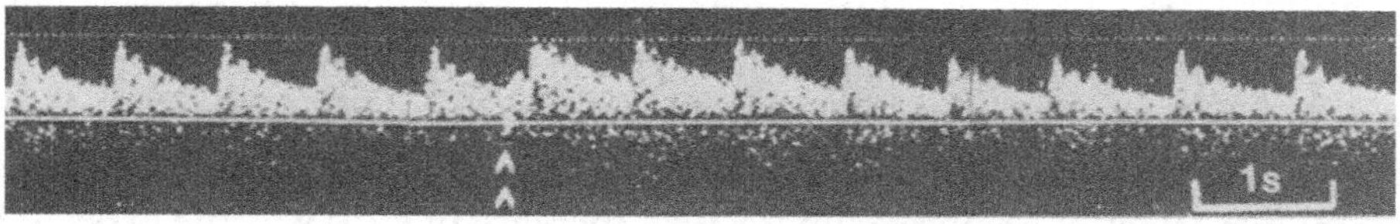

Fig. 3. Autoregulatory response of MCA velocity (flow) to a step decrease (arrowheads) of about 30 mm Hg in intracranial pressure. The CVR readjusts to new value within a few seconds

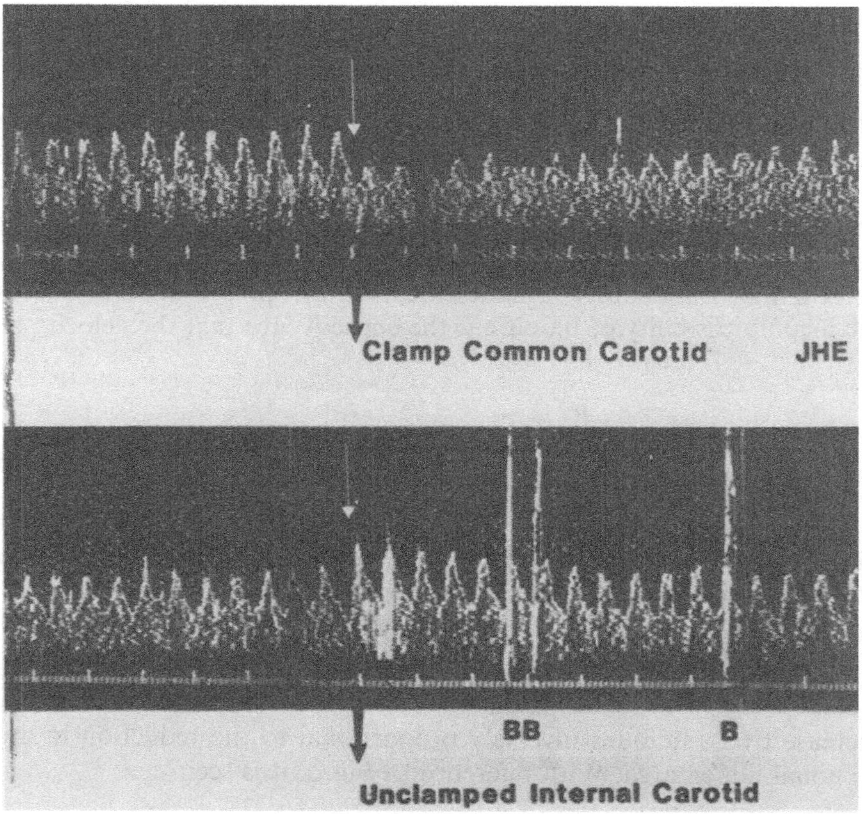

Fig. 4. Autoregulatory responses to 30 mm Hg decreases *upper* and increases *lower* in cerebral perfusion pressure during carotid surgery. Recording in ipsilateral MCA. Clamping and unclamping at arrows. Tick on zero-line indicate seconds. Sharp vertical artifacts in lower panel are probably caused by microemboli from the closed carotid. It is seen that the combination of collateral channels with cerebral autoregulation restores flow (velocity) after clamping

The pulsatile dynamics of the cerebrovascular bed is mainly governed by resistive, and less by compliance or "Windkessel" effects (see subsequent section) and it is therefore highly unlikely that the increases in V_{MCA} are caused by additional flow needed to fill up the compliant bed. The immediate effect of an approximate 30% increase in CPP was the expected proportional V_{MCA} increase. Filling up the compliance would have given an immediate high peak above this value which was not seen in the present recordings. The fact that V_{MCA} returned to control values (after 4 seconds) can only be explained by a rapid adjustment of the CVR.

Pressure Flow Relationship of Stenosis: The Bernoulli Effect

The linear viscous resistance of Poiseulle is responsible for the main energy loss in a vascular bed. The loss is caused by the viscous friction between layers of fluid. Normally, the velocity of flow decreases as the flow divides and enters into smaller and more numerous branches. In pathological circulatory states, local constriction of the flow in distributing arteries can cause a high *spatial* acceleration of the flow. The preservation of mass and the incompressibility of blood has the consequence that the velocity must

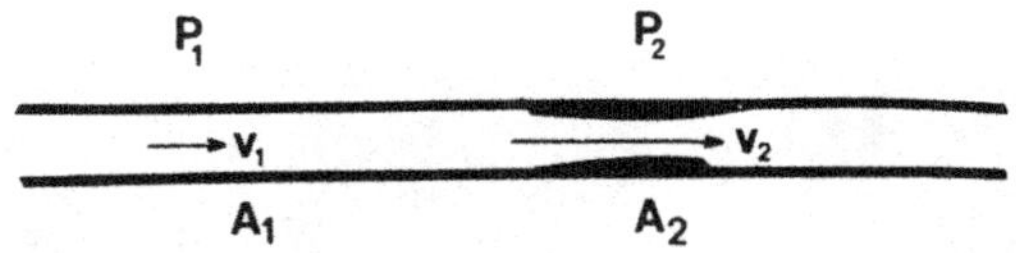

Fig. 5. The "continuity principle": P_1, v_1, A_1 pressure, velocity and cross-sectional area proximal to stenosis. P_2, v_2, A_2 same variables at the narrowest point in the stenotic channel

increase by an amount inversely proportional to the reduction in cross-sectional lumen area. With reference to Fig. 5. it is seen that:

$$A_1 V_1 = A_2 V_2$$

$$V_2 = V_1 A_1 / A_2 \quad (5)$$

At the entrance to the constriction, the blood must be accelerated. This acceleration is called spatial because the velocity increases as a function of space as the lumen narrows down. (This distinction is necessary to discriminate spatial acceleration from temporal which is caused by the pulsatile dynamics of the arterial flow.) Energy is involved in accelerating the fluid. To put it more precisely: during acceleration energy is converted from static (pressure) energy into kinetic energy. The conversion of energy was described by Bernoulli:

$$p_2 - p_1 = \triangle p = \frac{1}{2}\rho(V_2^2 - V_1^2) \tag{6}$$

$\triangle p$ is the pressure difference between the two points with velocity V_1 and V_2 respectively. ρ is the density of blood.

In the ideal situation, the kinetic energy would be converted back to pressure energy when the flow is decelerated distal to the stenosis. However, such recovery is not possible in practice (Berguer and Hwang 1974). The bruits and murmurs distal to a stenosis are manifestation of loss of energy into vortex formation and disturbed flow patterns. (The energy loss is strictly not a loss but rather a conversion to mostly thermal energy which does not help perfusion *per se*.)

The relationship between velocity and the pressure gradient described by Bernoulli is quite intriguing and involves only one other parameter—the density ρ which is known with a high degree of accuracy. When this formula was applied by Holen *et al.* (1976) in cardiology to estimate pressure differences or gradients noninvasively from Doppler data, they chose the mitral valve because the viscous losses would be negligible and the kinetic energy could not possibly be recovered inside the left ventricle. The correlation between measured and estimated pressure differences was good (Holen *et al.* 1976), and subsequent studies by other groups have confirmed this (Hatle *et al.* 1978).

In the cerebral circulation there are mainly three types of pathology which can cause high degrees of spatial acceleration:

1. Stenosis or arteriosclerotic lesions causing reduction in lumen area in carotid—or less frequently—in intracranial arteries.
2. Vasospasm due to contraction of vascular smooth muscle of intracranial arteries. This is a complication in subarachnoid hemorrhage, stroke, migraine, etc.
3. Involvement of relatively narrow communicating channels within the circle of Willis (ACoA, PCoA) in providing collateral flow (disease in the ipsilateral supply channels).

How much the Bernoulli loss (second power of velocity) and how much the linear Poiseulle loss each contributes in such circumstances has not been determined for typical stenotic/spastic lesions of cerebral arteries. However, when systolic velocities of 450 cm/sec have been found in spastic MCA's (unpublished data) the Bernoulli loss alone would give pressure differences of more than 70 mm Hg.

A graphic presentation of the combination of the properties of the two types of energy loss described above is shown in Fig. 6. Here it is assumed that neither the kinetic energy nor the impulse is recovered after the stenosis, so the curve thus represents the "worst-case" situation. Furthermore, it has been assumed that pre- and poststenotic velocities are low (< 100 cm/sec) so that their kinetic energies are minimal (<4 mm Hg).The different curves from bottom to top represent increasing viscous losses. In the physiological situation this can be interpreted as increasing length of the lesion, or

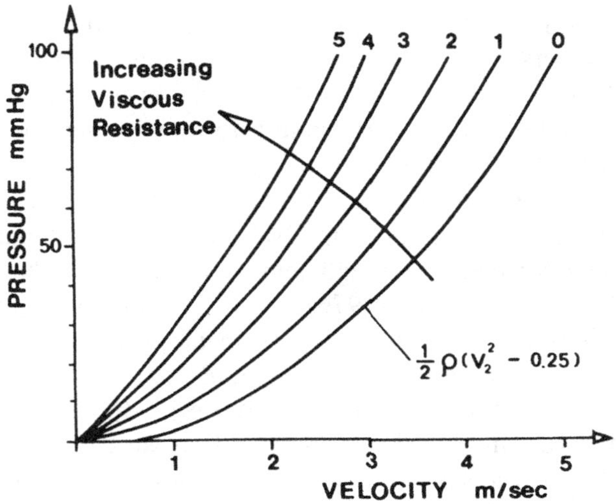

Fig. 6. Relationship of pressure drop over a stenosis to the jet velocity for different values of viscous resistance. Curve 0 represents kinetic losses only as found in mitral valve. Viscous resistance depends on length of stenosis, viscosity and the diameter and geometry of the lumen

increasing viscosity (hematocrit), or generally a smaller scale of the stenosis (smaller diameter, length and flow which leads to increasing viscous loss due to the fourth power of the radius in the Poiseulle equation).

At present it is too early to assign any of these curves to spasm or stenosis in the intracranial circulation. For stenosis of the human carotid bifurcation, scaled down *in vivo* experiments (dog abdominal aorta) indicate that the lower curve applies (Faccenda *et al.* 1985). Thus, there are reasons to hope that an estimate of pressure loss can be determined by Doppler velocity recordings from a stenosis. However, in extended cerebral vasospasm, the length of the constricted segment will play a more prominent role, and the pressure loss will certainly be greater than that predicted by the lower curve. Which of the upper curves applies to such situations is dependent on the extent of the spasm and the viscosity of the blood.

Transcranial Doppler for Evaluation of Intracranial Stenosis

Doppler ultrasound is widely recognized as an accurate noninvasive method for diagnosis of moderate to severe stenosis of the carotid bifurcation (Spencer and Reid 1979, Zwiebel *et al.* 1982, Lindegaard *et al.* 1984). Transcranial Doppler can be seen as an extension of these techniques to the intracranial circulation. The first preliminary report of intracranial Doppler for diagnosis of siphon disease came in 1983 (Spencer 1983). Stenotic lesions were characterized by high velocities and bruits, and basically similar criteria as for the carotid bifurcation were used in the evaluation. A recent report (Spencer and Whisler 1986) confirmed the accuracy of this method for detecting siphon lesions.

The transtemporal pathway has been used to evaluate stenosis of basal cerebral arteries (Lindegaard *et al.* 1986, Ringelstein *et al.* 1986), the hemodynamic principle of this approach being the same as that described by Aaslid *et al.* (1984) for evaluation of cerebrovascular spasm. Fig. 7 A shows the angiograms of a patient with severe (78%) stenosis of the middle cerebral artery. The Doppler findings, Fig. 8 A, were 250 cm/sec (time mean) in the stenosis, and distally a damped slow waveform (50 cm/sec systolic, 42 cm/sec mean) was recorded. At least a 25 mm Hg pressure loss can be expected (Fig. 6, lower curve). This lesion obviously had some hemodynamic effects.

Through the suboccipital approach, lesions of the basilar and intracranial vertebral arteries can be diagnosed. Fig. 7 B shows angiograms of a stenosis of the basilar artery. The Doppler recordings, Fig. 8 B, reveal a high velocity (178 cm/sec in systole, 122 cm/sec in mean), but the signals from both PCAs were essentially normal. The effect of this stenosis would be one of only moderate reduction in perfusion pressure according to one of the two lower curves of Fig. 6. The insignificant damping of the PCA waveform is a further indication of relatively small energy losses. However, it should be pointed out that semiquantitative determination of pressure loss from recordings such as these has to be confirmed by physiological experimental data.

The findings of one study (Lindegaard *et al.* 1982) are summarized in Fig. 9, in which the graph shows velocity as function of lumen dimension. (The data from the carotid siphon were obtained through the transorbital approach). The measurements of diameter were corrected for angiographic magnification. The findings were quite consistent with data reported from spasms of the MCA (Aaslid *et al.* 1984, see Fig. 1, Chapter 8, p. 120). The regression curve found in the spasm series is the broken line in Fig. 9. However, the deviations from the regression line seems to be greater in the spasm series than in the cases with stenosis. More data on intracranial stenosis are necessary before using statistical methods.

Lindegaard *et al.* (1986) also reported one case where the transcranial Doppler was used to diagnose an MCA occlusion. This is a technically difficult diagnosis to reach from Doppler data because: 1. The investigator must be sure there is indeed a transcranial window which could normally be used to identify an MCA signal. If this is the case then, 2. there is the additional difficulty in identifying Doppler signals in the absence of MCA flow which is used as a reference point in normal cases. The use of

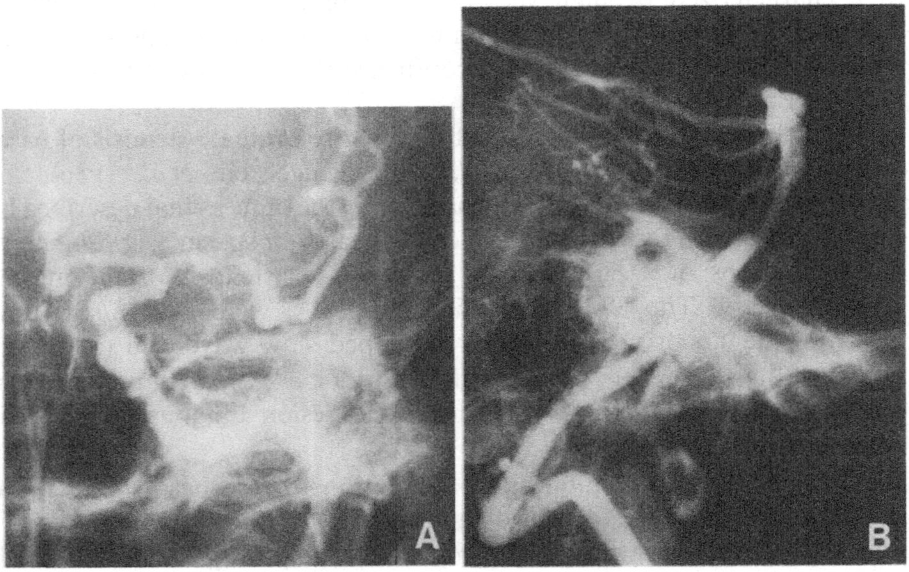

Fig. 7 A and B. *A* Angiogram of a patient with stenosis of the middle cerebral artery. Transcranial Doppler recordings show in Fig. 8 A. *B* Angiogram of patient with stenosis of the basilar artery. Transcranial Doppler recordings shown in Fig. 8 B. [From: Lindegaard K-F, Bakke SJ, Aaslid R, Nornes H (1986) Doppler diagnosis of intracranial artery occlusive disorders. J Neurol Psychiat (in press)]

transcranial Doppler for exploring MCA occlusion requires experience and good technical skill of the investigator. In the case referred to, other signals were found (ACA, PCA) on the side of the MCA occlusion, and the diagnosis was verified by CT scan and autopsy.

The neurovascular significance of transcranial Doppler diagnosis of intracranial atherosclerotic lesions can be summed up as follows:

1. If the extracranial Doppler and B-mode examination does not explain a patient's neurovascular symptoms (strokes and TIAs), the transcranial Doppler can explore the segments of the intracranial circulation that can be insonated from the different windows. In most patients this territory covers the siphon and the basal cerebral arteries where stenotic/occlusive lesions are found.

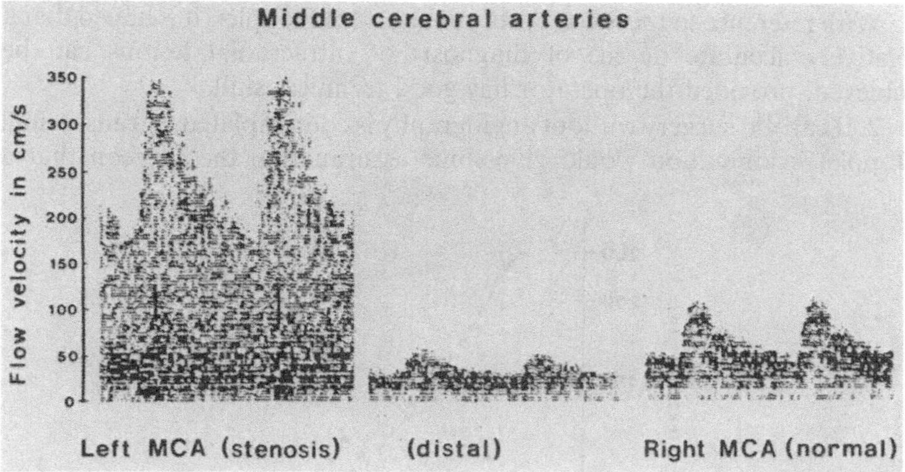

Fig. 8 A

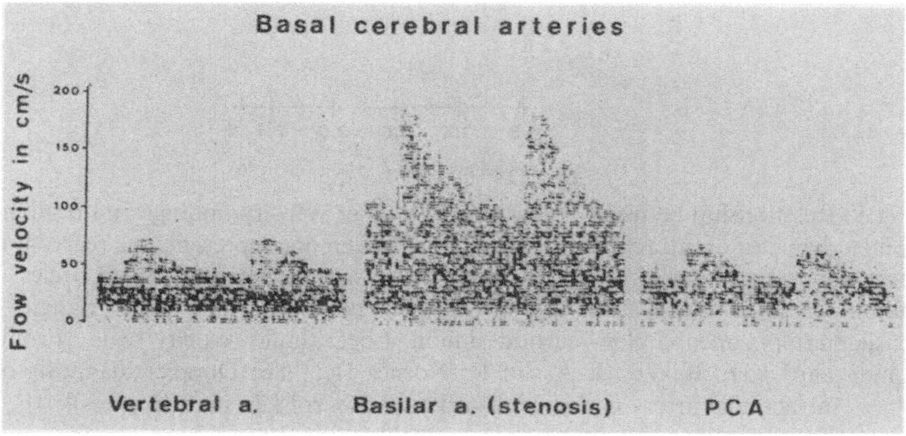

Fig. 8 B

Fig. 8 A and B. *A* Transcranial Doppler recordings from a patient with MCA stenosis on the left side (angiogram in Fig. 7 A). Right MCA velocities shown for comparison. *B* Transcranial Doppler recordings from a patient with basilar artery stenosis (angiogram in Fig. 7 B). The distal flow in the posterior cerebral artery (PCA) did not seem to be significantly affected even though the systolic flow velocity in the stenosis was close to 200 cm/sec. [From: Lindegaard K-F, Bakke S J, Aaslid R, Nornes H (1986) Doppler diagnosis of intracranial artery occlusive disorders. J Neurol Psychiat (in press)]

With reference to the few reports on this use of Doppler, it is hoped that a relatively accurate degree of diagnosis of intracranial lesions can be achieved, provided the operator has good technical skill.

2. If carotid surgery without angiography is contemplated, a transcranial Doppler examination would give some assurance to the surgeon that a

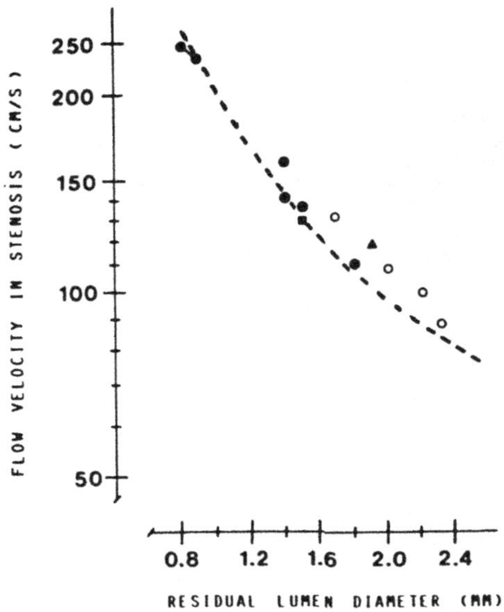

Fig. 9. Relationship between Transcranial Doppler velocity findings and residual lumen diameter of intracranial stenosis. The broken line represents the regression line found in a larger series on cerebral vasospasm (1). Symbols: Filled circles—middle cerebral artery; filled square—anterior cerebral artery; filled triangle—basilar artery; open circles—carotid siphon. Logarithmic velocity scale. [From: Lindegaard K-F, Bakke SJ, Aaslid R, Nornes H (1986) Doppler diagnosis of intracranial artery occlusive disorders. J Neurol Psychiat (in press)]

severe tandem lesion further upstream would not compromise the results of the endarterectomy.

3. The severity of the intracranial lesion can be evaluated (rather grossly at present, hopefully more accurately in the future) from velocity readings. This can give valuable information for the decision of whether an extra-intracranial bypass operation would be beneficial for the brain circulation of the patient or not. This factor may become even more important in the future as surgical skill becomes more refined. Then a corresponding improvement of the hemodynamic analysis of the lesion and the assessment of efficacy of shunting procedures in also needed (Harders 1985). Moreover, the noninvasive Doppler method is ideal for monitoring the individual course of the disease.

Collateral Flow in the Circle of Willis

Anatomic studies (Alpers *et al.* 1959), reveal that the circle of Willis is highly variable from one individual to another, with only 52% of the circles in their material being classified as normal. Twenty-seven percent of the circles had one or more string-like segments, and multiple anomalies were present in 13% of the series. If the ICA is severely stenosed or occluded, the supply of collateral flow to the affected hemisphere depends critically upon the patency of one or more collateral channels. The circle of Willis is probably a better collateral source than anastomoses with the external carotid artery, since the latter supply has to cross through long narrow arterial channels with considerable flow resistance, while the connections within the circle are relatively short. The variability of the anatomy of the circle of Willis is reflected in the variability of stump pressures (Sweet and Bennett 1948). Stump pressures can vary between individuals from as low as 10 mm Hg up to almost the level of the arterial blood pressure.

The resistance to flow in a given collateral circle connection is a mixture of a viscous linear component and a quadratic component (Fig. 6). The quadratic is mainly determined by vessel diameter, while the linear is a function of diameter, length and viscosity. Even if models may be useful to study the effects of different configurations of the circle on the distribution of flow, data from the individual patient is necessary for clinical decisions. The hemodynamics within segments of the circle of Willis during carotid clamping or compression were recorded by Nornes (1972, 1973), Nornes and Wikeby (1977) using electromagnetic flowmetry and by Nornes *et al.* (1979) and Gilsbach (Chapter 9) using intraoperative Doppler instrumentation.

Compression Tests

With the transcranial Doppler method it is now possible to record noninvasively the effects on flow within circle segments when the carotids are compressed. Such recording were reported by Aaslid *et al.* (1982). A further example is shown in Figs. 3 to 6 in the previous chapter (pp. 46–52). During CCA compression, the velocity in the contralateral ACA rose to 2.7 times the control value. Since volume flow is proportional to velocity, it would seem reasonable to assume that this channel now supplied both ACA territories, plus parts of the MCA territory. This was verified by recording from the ipsilateral ACA, where the velocity reversed to a value of 1.1 times the control value.

Fig. 6, p. 52, shows that velocity in the ipsilateral PCA increased to 1.4 times control, which means that the PCoA also supplied collateral flow to the MCA. Such tests not only show that communicating arteries are open, but also give semiquantiative information on the capacity of the different channels. Transcranial Doppler and compression tests would seem a rational procedure when ligation of the ICA is contemplated, or where the surgeon needs information on collateral sources in planning carotid surgery when shunting would be difficult or impossible.

There is a need for a physiological complement to the anatomical studies referred to at the start of this section to determine how the capacities of the different circle pathways vary within the normal population. Such a study could now be carried out with the aid of the transcranial Doppler as described above.

Patients with Chronic Lesions

In a study on an series of 77 patients with stenosis or occlusion of the carotid bifurcation, Lindegaard *et al.* (1985) used transcranial Doppler to evaluate collateral flow. In 31 of these patients, angiography demonstrated cross-over flow to the MCA on the side with the most severe lesion. Reversed ACA flow could be shown with transcranial Doppler in 29 of these cases. Moreover, the contralateral side had significantly increased ACA velocity (greater than 1.5 times the velocity in the MCA on that side) in 26 of these cases, and the remaining 5 cases all had ACA velocities between 1.25 and 1.5 of those of the MCA.

In 30 patients there was collateral filling of the MCA from the PCA. In 19 of these, the velocity in the PCA was above 1.5 times of the ipsilateral MCA, 7 were within 1.2 to 1.5 times the MCA and the remaining 4 PCAs were within 1 to 1.25 times of their respective MCAs. In the normal subject the PCA velocity is usually much lower than that of the MCA. (See previous chapter on normal values.) The high collateral flow velocities reported in these two subseries reflect increased perfusion territory and increased demand for blood flow of channels not normally dimensioned for these flow loads.

The transcranial Doppler findings in a patient with occlusion of the left ICA and 90% stenosis of the right are shown in Fig. 10 (note that the ACA signals shown below the zero-line represent flow away from the probe). The bilaterally augmented PCA velocity indicated collateral supply from the posterior circulation. Furthermore, the absence of signals from the left ACA in combination with the augmented velocity in the right ACA (compared to the MCA on that side) indicate collateral flow through the ACoA, and that both distal ACAs were supplied from the right side.

Another case with unilateral (left ICA) occlusion and no stenosis is presented in Fig. 11. Retrograde velocities in the left ACA and highly augmented velocities in the right ACA were indicative of a good crossover filling via the anterior part of the circle of Willis.

The information that can be obtained from such studies complements

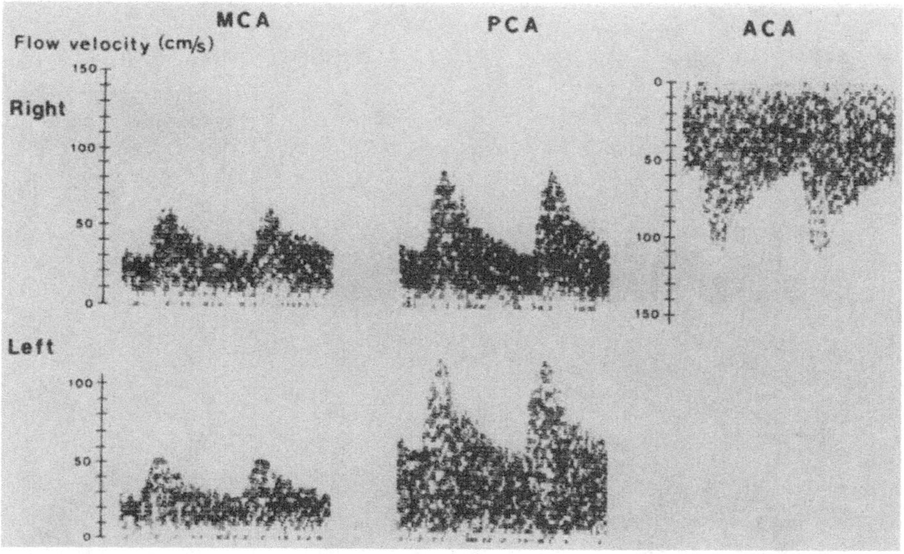

Fig. 10. Transcranial Doppler findings in a 66 year-old man in whom right carotid angiography revealed 90% stensosis of the extracranial internal carotid artery (ICA) and proximal anterior cerebral artery (ACA) filling the right and left pericallosal arteries (distal ACAs) only. Left carotid angiography showed total ICA occlusion, and vertebral angiography demonstrated left middle cerebral artery (MCA) filling through a collateral channel from the left posterior cerebral artery (PCA) but no filling of the left ACA. The velocity in the left PCA, (V_{PCA}) was 2.0 times the left V_{MCA} indicating collateral flow. The right V_{ACA} was 1.7 of the right V_{MCA}. No Doppler signals were found from the left ACA. The pulsatile indices and velocities for the MCAs were approximately equal, with reference to the PCA waveform the pulsatility transmission index (PTI) was 0.73 right and 0.72 left. [From Lindegaard K-F, Bakke SJ, Grolimund P, Aaslid R, Huber P, Nornes H (1985) Assessment of intracranial hemodynamics in carotid artery disease by transcranial Doppler ultrasound. J Neurosurg 63: 890–898, with permission]

that from extracranial Doppler and B-mode images of the carotid bifurcation to give a more complete noninvasive picture of the hemodynamic state of the cerebral circulation in patients with significant disease of the carotid bifurcation. In the next section we shall consider the pulsatile dynamics of flow in these arteries and how an analysis of waveforms can add even more information.

Pulsatile Dynamics: The Contribution of the Cerebral "Windkessel"

The effects discussed above can be described as static pressure flow relationship which means that the flow (or the velocity) is a function of the instantaneous cerebral perfusion pressure only and not of the prehistory of the waveforms. Dynamic pressure-flow relationships mean that some the

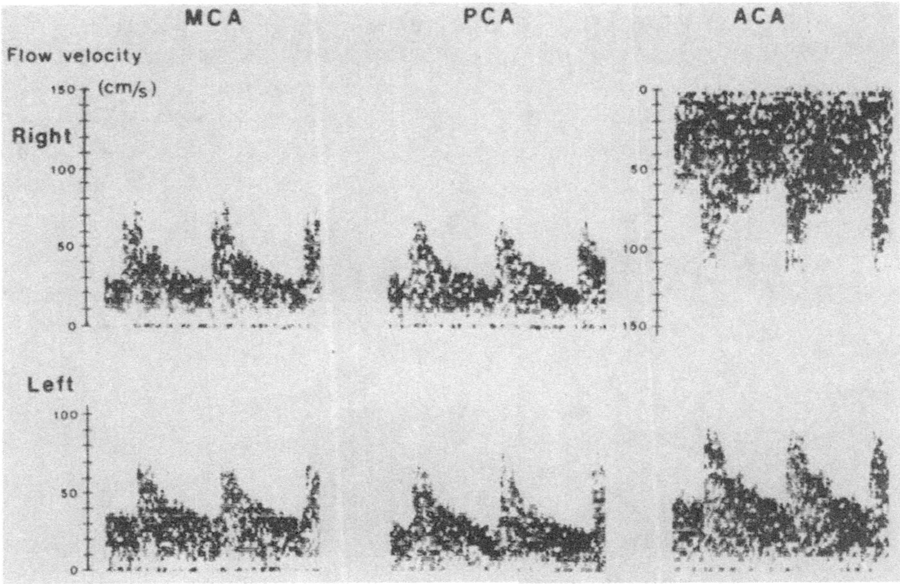

Fig. 11. Transcranial Doppler findings in a 58-year-old man in whom left carotid angiography confirmed total internal carotid artery (ICA) occlusion. Right carotid angiography revealed no ICA stenosis but did indicate collateral fillings across the midline into the left middle cerebral artery (MCA), and the vertebral angiograms were normal with no filling of collateral vessels. Collateral flow over the anterior circle of Willis is indicated in the spectral display by retrograde flow velocities in the left anterior cerebral artery (ACA) and an augmented (1.75 times the V_{MCA}) velocity in the right ACA. Both posterior cerebral arteries (PCAs) demonstrated lower Doppler shifts than the MCAs indicating that they did not function as collateral supply sources. The left MCA demonstrated reduced pulsatility transmission index (PTI = 0.76), but the absolute velocity was not reduced compared to the right side. [From Lindegaard K-F, Bakke SJ, Grolimund P, Aaslid R, Huber P, Nornes H (1985) Assessment of intracranial hemodynamics in carotid artery disease by transcranial Doppler ultrasound. J Neurosurg 63: 890–898, with permission)

previous history of the time course of the variables is needed in order to describe the present state. When pulsatile hemodynamics is considered, the most important dynamic relationship is the "Windkessel" effect.

The simple fact that the arterial pressure normally pulsates between 75 and 120 mm Hg in spite of the intermittent ejection from the left ventricle is due to the elasticity of the arterial system acting as a reservoir of the energy supplied during systole. A so-called "Windkessel", where the pressure is a function of the *integrated* net flow into the reservoir can describe the main shape of the arterial or aortic pressure waveform (Frank 1899):

$$ABP = F\left(\int^{t} (\text{inflow-outflow})\, dt\right) \qquad (7)$$

The function F (.) is in its simplest form the static relationship between volume (= the time integral of net inflow) and the pressure in the arterial system. A typical pressure volume relationship is shown in Fig. 12 left. The slope of this curve is called arterial volume compliance C = dV/dp. The curve is not linear: the compliance decreases with increasing arterial pressure.

While the necessity of including this property when describing aortic pressure is obvious, it is not so evident that it plays a significant role in the cerebral circulation where the Doppler signals are typically representative of low resistance flow. However, in many cases of pathology, the

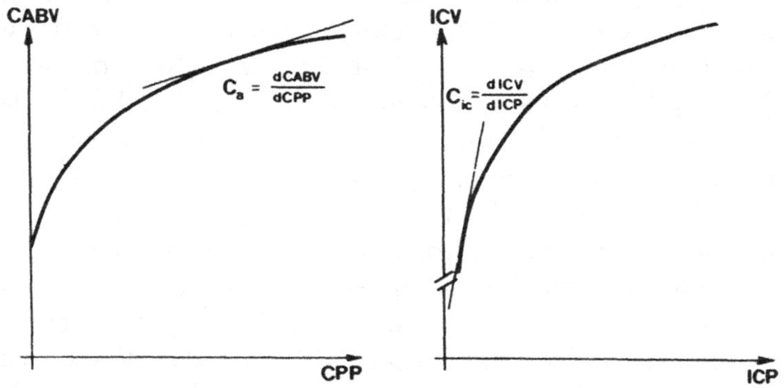

Fig. 12. Pressure-volume relationship of cerebral arteries and arterioles *left* and the intracranial space *right*. *CPP* cerebral perfusion pressure; *CABV* cerebral arterial blood volume; *ICP* intracranial pressure; *ICV* intracranial volume; C_a volume compliance of cerebral arteries and arterioles; C_{ic} compliance of intracranial cavity

compliance effect explains the waveform changes. Also, in the normal state the Frankian Windkessel is certainly there—but its effects are masked by the influence of the low cerebral vascular resistance.

The ordinate in Fig. 12 left is transmural pressure which is equal to ABP-ICP or, as defined above, cerebral perfusion pressure CPP. In addition, the intracranial space has its own pressure-volume relationship (Fig. 12, right). An incremental increase in cerebral arterial blood volume, dCABV, also represents an additional volume added to the total intracranial volume, and gives an addition dICP to the intracranial pressure. Any incremental pulsation in the arterial blood pressure, dABP, will be shared between two different compartments: dABP = dCPP + dICP. Linearizing the pressure-volume curves we find:

$$\begin{aligned} dCABV &= (dABP - dICP)\ C_a \\ &= dABP - CABV\ C_a/C_{ic} \\ &= dABP/(1/C_a + 1/C_{ic}) \end{aligned} \tag{8}$$

When the intracranial pressure increases, the arteries become more elastic (increasing C_a) and the intracranial space becomes stiffer (decreasing C_{ic})—thus the pressure-volume relationship is shifted from arterial compartment to the total pressure-volume relationship of the intracranial space.

There are different situations when the effect of compliance markedly effects the flow (or velocity) waveform:

1. A proximal stenosis (carotid artery) leads to a damped velocity waveform (Gosling and King 1974, Lindegaard *et al.* 1985). Because of the increased inflow resistance, the "Windkessel" fills up more slowly and the effect is a more rounded inflow waveshape with less pulsatility.
2. Decreased pulsatility has also been observed in arteriovenous malformation feeders (pp. 94–95). This is probably due to the very low flow resistance in conjunction with high volume stiffness of the AVM.
3. Increased flow velocity pulsatility is observed during decreased arterial pCO_2 (hyperventilation) as described by Markwalder *et al.* (1984). The hypocapnic state causes an increased flow resistance, thereby unmasking the "Windkessel" effect.
4. Abnormally increased intracranial pressure gives rise to a very pulsatile waveform (Chapter 10, pp. 157–158) which was described by Greenfield and Tindall (1965). Two factors can be hypothesized to explain this phenomenon: The pulsatility of the CPP increases with increasing ICP, Fig. 1; and secondly, the total volume compliance increases so that more blood is required in systole to fill the "Windkessel".

Pulsatility Analysis in Patients with Carotid Artery Disease

For the analysis of cerebral hemodynamics in patients with carotid occlusive disease, the damping effect 1) described above is the most important. Theoretically, the relationship between the shape of the waveform and the total parallel resistance of stenotic/collateral channels is quite complicated. The initial study by Lindegaard *et al.* (1985) used the pulsatility index defined by Gosling (1974):

$$PI = (Vs - Vd)/Vm \tag{9}$$

Vs, Vd and Vm are peak systolic, end diastolic and time mean velocities respectively. This formula was proposed for use in peripheral vessels, where in the normal resting state, "Windkessel" effects dominate over resistance effects. The arterial pulsewave is *transmitted* or *propagated* through the vascular tree and changes in the waveform occur when it has to pass through an arterial narrowing with a significant flow resistance. To improve the sensitivity of the PI, one can therefore compare the waveform at a selected site (MCA on ipsilateral side) with a waveform assumed to be propagated through a nonstenosed channel. A pulsatility *transmission* index (essentially a normalized pulsatility index) has the purpose of minimizing the influence of the particular shape of the driving pressure waveform on the index:

$$PTI = PI/PIref \tag{10}$$

PI is the Gosling pulsatility index in the artery being studied, PIref is the corresponding index in a reference artery without any proximal flow obstruction. For normal subjects, the PI in the right MCA was used as PIref. The PTI for the left MCA was 0.995 ± 0.04 (mean $\pm$ standard deviation) in 40 subjects without carotid artery or intracranial disease. A PTI of 0.92 would be 2 standard devations from the normal, and has been proposed as a useful clinical limit for detecting cases where there are significant lesions in the supply arteries (Lindegaard *et al.* 1985). In such cases, the PIref is defined as highest pulsatility index for either the MCAs or the PCAs. This will normally be found on the opposite side of the most severe lesion. Figs. 10 and 11 describes the PTI findings for two patients.

For a total of 81 patient hemispheres with stenosis $> 75\%$, (bilateral lesions included) the PTI was below 0.92 in all cases except 3. All PTI values from patients with stenosis less than 40% were above 0.92.

The PTI is predominantly a function of *total* inflow resistance, the great variation in the collaterals explaining the wide range in PTI observed in patients with occlusions. An index based on side differences in Doppler recordings of mean velocity would miss all cases where the cerebral autoregulation can cope with the loss in perfusion pressure caused by the lesion. In contrast, the autoregulatory vasodilation acts to increase the sensitivity of the PTI because the effect of decreased peripheral vascular resistance is decreased pulsatility.

Future Possibilities in Pulsatility Waveform Analysis

More exact and refined methods of analyzing pulse-wave dynamics can be employed if a computer is available for the data processing. The classic way of analyzing periodic waveforms is Fourier analysis. The arterial pressure, flow and velocity waveforms do exhibit periodicity with a basic frequency equal to the heart rate. The waveform can be analyzed with respect to the relative contribution of the different Fourier coefficients (Woodcock *et al.* 1972). The application of Fourier analyses is shown in Fig. 13 for a V_{MCA} waveform recording. The upper panel shows the spectra, the gray trace in the lower panel is the spectral outline. The white trace is the pulsatile signal reconstructed from the Fourier coefficients. For the first (left) beat, only one harmonic is used in the reconstruction, resulting in a sinewave with an offset. The second beat shows the result of using two harmonics. For the third and fourth beat, three and five harmonics are used respectively. The amplitudes of the Fourier coefficients for each of these harmonics is shown by the printout between the two panels. It is seen that increasing the number of coefficients gives a better reproduction of the original waveform—five harmonics actually give a very good fit to the original curve.

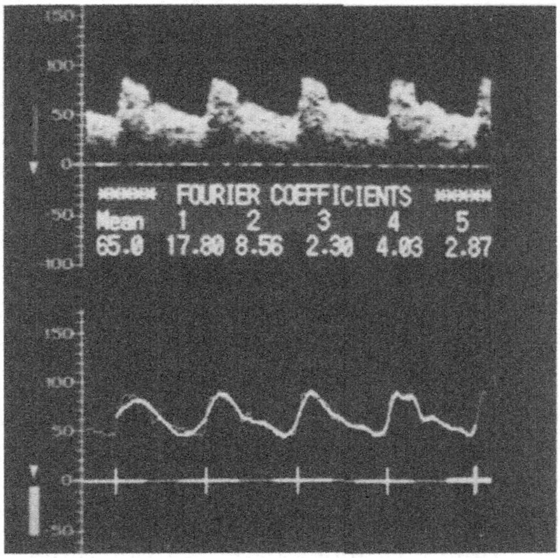

Fig. 13. Fourier analysis of MCA velocity waveform *upper* panel shows raw spectra. *Lower panel* shows gray tracing—outline of spectra; white tracing (partly covering gray tracing)—representation of waveform using *1, 2, 3, or 5* harmonics (successive beats)

This type of analysis was used in an attempt reported by Aaslid *et al.* (1985) to relate the pulsatility of the V_{MCA} to the cerebral perfusion pressure in a group of 10 patients undergoing ventricular infusion tests for determination of CSF fluid dynamics. The first harmonic, ABP_1, of the arterial blood pressure was also used in the formula:

$$CPP_{index} = ABP_1 \cdot V_{MCA\,0}/V_{MCA\,1} \tag{11}$$

The advantage of using only first harmonics (ABP_1, $V_{MCA\,1}$) and mean ($V_{MCA\,0}$) in the calculations is to avoid the influence of the higher harmonics of the pressure pulse. These are propagated in the arterial tree with significant distortion (O'Rourke 1970). The amplitude of the first harmonic is practically equal in the arm and in the aorta. The cerebral circulation has shorter transmission line than the arm so the first harmonic of pressure will be even less distorted there. The results from this series show good correlation ($r = 0.89$) between the CPPindex and the real CPP. The regression line was $CPP = 1.1\ CPP_{index} - 5$ mm Hg.

The purpose of using such advanced methods of pulsatility analysis is to improve the quantitative accuracy of transcranial Doppler recordings for intracranial and perfusion pressure estimation as compared with what can be achieved by more conventional approaches (Chapter 10).

References

1. Aaslid R, Huber P, Nornes H (1984) Evaluation of cerebrovascular spasm with transcranial Doppler ultrasound. J Neurosurg 60: 37–41
2. Aaslid R, Markwalder T-M, Nornes H (1982) Noninvasive transcranial Doppler ultrasound recording of flow velocity in basal cerebral arteries. J Neurosurg 57: 769–774.
3. Aaslid R, Nornes H (1984) Musical murmurs in human cerebral arteries after subarachnoid hemorrhage. J Neurosurg 60: 32–36
4. Aaslid R, Lundar T, Lindegaard K-F, Nornes H (1986) Estimation of cerebral perfusion pressure from arterial blood pressure and transcranial Doppler recordings. In: Teasdale G, Brock M (eds) Intracranial pressure 6. Springer, Berlin Heidelberg New York
5. Alpers BJ, Berry RG, Paddison RM (1959) Anatomical studies of the circle of Willis in normal brain. AMA Arch Neurol Psychiat 81: 25–34
6. Berguer R, Hwang NHC (1974) Critical stenosis: A theoretical and experimental solution. Ann Surg: 39–50
7. Bullock R, Mendelow AD, Bone I, Patterson J, Macleod WN, Allardice G (1981) Cerebral blood flow and CO_2 responsiveness as an indicator of collateral reserve capacity in patients with carotid arterial disease. Br J Surg 72: 348–351
8. Faccenda F, Usui Y, Spencer M (1985) Doppler measurement of the pressure drop caused by arterial stenosis: An experimental study: A case report. Angiology 4: 899–905
9. Fog M (1937) Cerebral circulation. The reaction of the pial arteries to a fall in blood pressure. Arch Neurol Psych 37: 351–364
10. Frank O (1899) Die Grundform des arteriellen Pulses. Z Biol 37: 483–526
11. Fry DL, Thomas LJ, Greenfield JC Jr (1980) Flow in collapsable tubes. In: Patel DJ, Vaishnav RN (eds) Basic hemodynamics and its role in disease processes. University Park Press, Baltimore
12. Gosling RG, King DH (1974) Continuous wave ultrasound as an alternative and complement to X-rays in vascular examinations. In: Reneman RE (ed) Cardiovascular applications of ultrasound. North-Holland, Amsterdam, pp 266–282
13. Greenfield JC, Tindall GT (1965) Effect of acute increase in intracranial pressure on blood flow in the internal carotid artery. J Clin Invest 44: 1343–1351
14. Halpern W, Osol G (1985) Influence of transmural pressure on myogenic responses of isolated cerebral arteries of the rat. Biomed Eng 13: 287–294

15. Harders A, Gilsbach JM (1985) Transcranial Doppler sonography and its application in extracranial-intracranial bypass surgery. Neurol Res 7: 129–141
16. Hatle L, Brubakk AO, Tromsdal A, Angelsen BAJ (1978) Noninvasive assessement of pressure drop in mitral stenosis by Doppler ultrasound. Br Heart J 40: 131–140
17. Holen J, Aaslid R, Landmark K, Simonsen S (1976) Determination of pressure gradient in mitral stenosis with a noninvasive ultrasound Doppler technique. Acta Med Scand 199: 455–460
18. Johnson PC (1980) The myogenic response. Handbook of physiology—The cardiovascular system II, 2: 409–443
19. Knowlton PF, Starling EH (1912) The influence of variations in temperature and blood pressure on the performance of the isolated mammalian heart. J Physiol 44: 206
20. Kontos HA, Wei EP, Navari RM, Levasseur JE, Rosenblum WI, Patterson JL (1978) Responses of cerebral arteries and arterioles to acute hypotension and hypertension. Am J Physiol 234: H371–383
21. Lindegaard K-F, Bakke SJ, Grolimund P, Aaslid R, Huber P, Nornes H (1985) Assessment of intracranial hemodynamics in carotid artery disease by transcranial Doppler ultrasound. J Neurosurg 63: 890–898
22. Lindegaard K-F, Bakke SJ, Aaslid R, Nornes H (1986) Doppler diagnosis of intracranial artery occlusive disorders. J Neurol Psychiat (in press)
23. Lindegaard K-F, Bakke SJ, Grip A, Nornes H (1984) Pulsed Doppler techniques for measuring instantaneous maximum and mean flow velocities in carotid arteries. Ultrasound Med Biol 10: 419–426
24. Lindegaard K-F, Grip A, Nornes H (1980) Precerebral haemodynamics in brain tamponade. Neurochirurgia 23: 133–142
25. Lundar T, Lindegaard K-F, Fröysaker T, Aaslid R, Wiberg J, Nornes H (1985) Cerebral perfusion during nonpulsatile cardiopulmonary bypass. Ann Thorac Surg: 40: 144–150
26. Lundar T, Lindegaard K-F, Fröysaker T, *et al.* (1986) Dissociation between cerebral autoregulation and CO_2 reactivity during nonpulsatile cardiopulmonary bypass. Ann Thorac Surg 40 (in press)
27. Markwalder TM, Grolimund P, Seiler R, Roth F, Aaslid R (1984) Dependency of blood flow velocity in the middle cerebral artery on end-tidal carbon dioxide partial pressure—A transcranial Doppler study. J Cerebr Blood Flow Metab 4: 368–372
28. Naratomi H, Meyer JS, Sakai F, Yamaguchi F, Shaw T (1979) Effects of advancing age on regional blood flow. Arch Neurol 36: 410–416
29. Nornes H (1972) Hemodynamic aspects in the management of carotid-cavernous fistula. J Neurosurg 37: 687–694
30. Nornes H (1973) The role of the circle of Willis in graded occlusion of the internal carotid artery in man. Acta Neurochir 28: 165–177
31. Nornes H, Grip A, Wikeby P (1979) Intraoperative evaluation of cerebral hemodynamics using Doppler technique. J Neurosurg 50: 570–577
32. Nornes H, Magnaes B, Aaslid R (1975) Observations in intracranial pressure plateau waves. In: Lundberg N, Ponten U, Brock M (eds), Intracranial pressure 2. Springer, Berlin Heidelberg New York, pp 421–426

33. Nornes H, Wikeby P (1977) Cerebral arterial blood flow dynamics. J Neurosurg 47: 810–818
34. O'Rourke M F (1970) Influence of ventricular ejection on the relationship between central aortic and brachial pressure pulse in man. Cardiovas Res 4: 291–300
35. Reneman RS, Arts T (1985) Dynamic capacitance of epicardial coronary arteries in vivo. J Biomech Eng 107: 29–33
36. Ringelstein EB, Korbmacher G, Zeumer H (1984) Detection of intracranial arterial lesions by means of a new transcranial Doppler device. Proceedings, application of Doppler ultrasound in medicine, Duesseldorf
37. Rittgers SE, Thornhill BM, Barnes RW (1983) Quantitative analysis of carotid artery Doppler spectral waveforms: Diagnostic value of parameters. Ultrasound in Med Biol 9: 255–264
38. Sekhar LN, Wasserman JF (1984) Noninvasive dedection of intracranial vascular lesions using an electronic stethoscope. J Neurosurg 60: 553–559
39. Spencer MP (1983) Intracranial carotid artery diagnosis with transorbital pulsed wave (PW) and continuous wave (CW) Doppler ultrasound. J Ultrasound in Med [Suppl] 2: 61
40. Spencer MP, Reid JM (1979) Quantification of carotid stenosis with continuous-wave Doppler ultrasound. Stroke 10: 326–330
41. Spencer MP, Whisler GD (1986) Transorbital Doppler diagnosis of intracranial arterial stenosis. Stroke (in press)
42. Strandgaard S, Paulson OB (1984) Cerebral autoregulation. Stroke 15: 413–416
43. Stromberg DD, Fox JR (1972) Pressure in the pial arterial microcirculation of the cat during changes in systemic arterial blood pressure. Circ Res 31: 229–239
44. Symon L, Held K, Dorsch NWC (1973) A study of regional autoregulation in the cerebral circulation to increased perfusion pressure in normocapnia and hypercapnia. Stroke 4: 139–147
45. Sweet WH, Bennett HS (1948) Changes in internal carotid pressure during carotid and jugular occlusion and their clinical significance. J Neurosurg 5: 178–195
46. Winn HR, Rubio R, Berne RM (1979) Brain adenosine production in the rat during 60 seconds of ischemia. Circ Res 45: 486–492
47. Woodcock JP, Gosling RG, Fitzgerald DE (1972) A new noninvasive technique for assessment of superficial femoral artery obstruction. Br J Surg 59: 226–231
48. Zwiebel WJ, Zagzebski JA, Crummy AB, Hirschner M (1982) Correlation of peak Doppler frequency with lumen narrowing in carotid stenosis. Stroke 13: 386–391

Authors' address: Dr. R. Aaslid, Institute of Applied Physiology and Medicine, 701 16th Avenue, Seattle, WA 98122, U.S.A.

6. Cerebral Arteriovenous Malformations

K.-F. Lindegaard, R. Aaslid, and *H. Nornes*

An arteriovenous malformation (AVM) is a development anomaly that results when the embryonic vascular network fails to evolve normally. Primarily normal arteries and veins are involved in conveying flow to and from the AVM [8]. Arteries leading to an AVM convey blood through the shunt and into the venous side. The size and flow rates of these arteries is far out of proportion to the low metabolism within an AVM. We therefore use the term "feeders" to distinguish these vessels from normal arteries purely conveying nutrient flow to neural tissues.

Angiographic investigation of patients with AVM provides essential anatomical information. The hemodynamic information concealed in an angiographic series may nevertheless be difficult to interpret. Methods to elucidate individual hemodynamic states are therefore clinically relevant.

The transcranial Doppler technique permits noninvasive recordings of blood flow velocity in basal cerebral arteries in adult individuals [2, 12]. The feeder arteries of cerebral AVMs are totally or partially within the range of this method. In the present study, the velocity and waveform pulsatility of AVM feeders and remote normal arteries were also compared to findings in healthy volunteers.

Clinical Doppler Investigation

Recording Techniques

Pulsed wave range-gated 2 MHz Doppler instruments with acoustical focusing and real-time spectrum analysis were used. The procedure and reference values for recording from the distal extracranial segment of the internal carotid arteries and from basal intracranial arteries have been described elsewhere [2, 12]. Flow velocities were measured as being the time-mean value of the Doppler velocity spectrum outline. The Doppler pulsatiliy index (PI) of the velocity spectrum outline (systolic velocity minus diastolic velocity divided by the time-mean value) was used to further characterize each recording [5, 12]. All values were the average from ten consecutive cardiac cycles.

Normal Individuals

Flow velocity and pulsatility in intracranial arteries varies considerably among individuals. In a series of healthy volunteers aged from 20 to 35 years we found middle cerebral artery (MCA) flow velocity to be 67 ± 7 cm/sec (mean and standard deviation) with Doppler pulsatility index (PI) values of 0.71 ± 0.10 [12].

In one individual, however, comparison of MCA flow velocity on opposing sides (relative flow velocity) showed a variation of $100 \pm 12\%$ (mean and standard deviation). The relative pulsatility index, designated pulsatility transmission index (PTI), showed even less intra-individual variation, $100 \pm 4\%$ [12].

Patients

Transcranial Doppler recordings from 16 patients with cerebral AVM were correlated with findings from selective cathether angiography.

The diameter of the AVM proper was measured from angiographic films. Two patients had a small AVM (diameter < 2 cm). Seven patients had a medium-size AVM (diameter ranging from about 2 to about 4 cm, and seven patients had a large AVM (over 4 cm).

The results of angiography and Doppler investigation were interpreted independently. The Wilcoxon rank test for two samples was used for statistical evaluation of differences.

Differentiation Between AVM Feeders and Normal Arteries

In principle, the resistance to flow through an AVM is low. It is therefore possible to diagnose AVMs and to locate individual AVM feeder arteries from findings of flow velocity and waveform pulsatility outside the ranges for expected variation.

The MCA contralateral to the AVM represented normal remote arteries in 15 patients. Recordings from the posterior cerebral artery (PCA) were used for this purpose in one patient with a large midline AVM fed by both MCAs. The flow velocity levels in normal remote arteries were from 49 to 80 cm/sec, median: 66 cm/sec. with Doppler pulsatility index (PI) from 0.66 to 1.10, median: 0.90. These values are within the ranges previously demonstrated in healthy volunteers [12].

The difference between AVM feeders and normal remote arteries in the individual patients was usually apparent immediately from the real-time spectral display (Figs. 1 and 2) and from listening to the Doppler audio signal. Recordings from intracranial arteries shown angiographically as feeding medium or large-size AVMs, showed flow velocity levels from 54 to

200 cm/sec, median: 112 cm/sec with PI values from 0.30 to 0.74, median: 0.55. Relative velocities were from 0.81 to 3.77, median: 1.65, with PTI from 0.33 to 0.94, median: 0.65. No significant difference was found between large and medium-size AVMs.

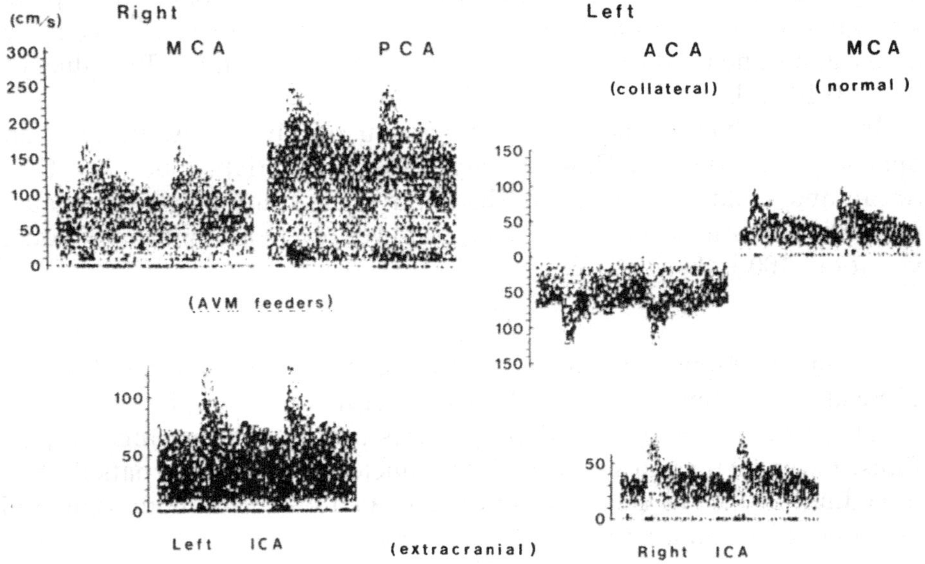

Fig. 1. Doppler recordings from man, 24 years. Large AVM right parietal region. Right middle cerebral artery (MCA) has flow velocity of 126 cm/sec with pulsatility index 0.53. Right posterior cerebral artery (PCA) had flow velocity 202 cm/sec with PI 0.38. These flow velocity patterns are characteristic of AVM feeder arteries. Left MCA flow velocity is 52 cm/sec with PI 1.10, typical of remote normal arteries. Left anterior cerebral artery (ACA) had a normal flow direction, but high velocity, 104 cm/sec, with PI 0.70, indicating its role as a feeder collateral into the opposite carotid territory. Sampling depth for recordings from MCA: 45 mm, PCA: 65 mm, ACA: 60 mm. Extracranial Doppler recordings (lower) showed very high flow velocity, 82 cm/sec, in the right internal carotid artery (ICA). Flow velocity in left ICA was 46 cm/sec. Sampling depth for ICA recordings was 45 mm, using same equipment as for transcranial investigation

Theoretically, 95% of normal individuals are contained within two standard deviations from the mean value. We therefore considered as pathological all findings outside of 2 SDs from the previously established reference mean values.

Using these criteria for relative flow velocity and for PTI, the diagnosis of AVM was obtained from transcranial Doppler investigation in all 14 patients with medium or large AVM. A striking, inverse relationship between relative flow velocity and PTI was seen when comparing recordings from different vessels in the individual patient (Fig. 4). However, transcranial Doppler investigation was false negative in the two patients with small AVM (diameter <2 cm).

Used as the only diagnostic criterion, absolute flow velocity was false negative in 4 of the 31 angiographically documented feeder arteries, yielding

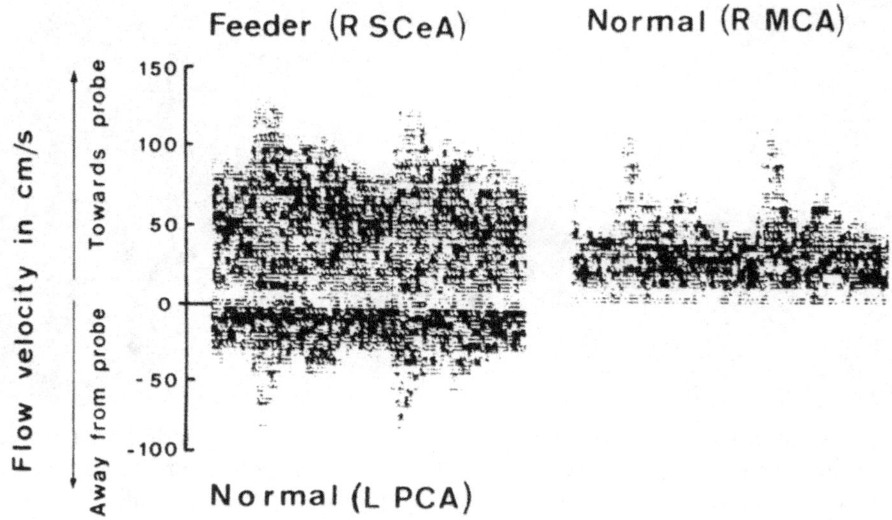

Fig. 2. Transcranial Doppler recordings in man, 42 years, with symptoms and signs of subarachnoid hemorrhage. Velocity pattern recorded from the right middle cerebral artery (MCA) was within normal range. Signals recorded in the expected location of the right posterior cerebral artery (PCA) showed high velocities, 98 cm/sec with PI 0.58. The left PCA could be recorded simultaneously, showing velocity waveforms within normal range. This permitted the diagnosis of an AVM. Angiographically, the AVM feeder artery proved to be the right superior cerebellar artery (Fig. 3 D)

a sensitivity of 87%. Relative flow velocity was also false negative in 4 feeders (sensitivity 83%). This reflects the well-known fact that AVM feeder arteries dilate in response to the high volume flow. The resulting flow velocity increase is therefore less than expected.

Absolute PI values proved of limited value in diagnosing AVMs, being false negative in 16 of the 31 feeders. In one patient with a large AVM, as well as in 5 of the 7 patients with a medium-size AVM, the use of PI alone would not have permitted the diagnosis of an AVM at all (sensitivity 50%). This was clearly a consequence of the wide PI range seen even among healthy individuals. However, the PTI indicated a correct diagnosis in the 29 feeders supplying medium or large AVMs (sensitivity 93%). The sensitivity for identifying individual patients as having an AVM was 87%.

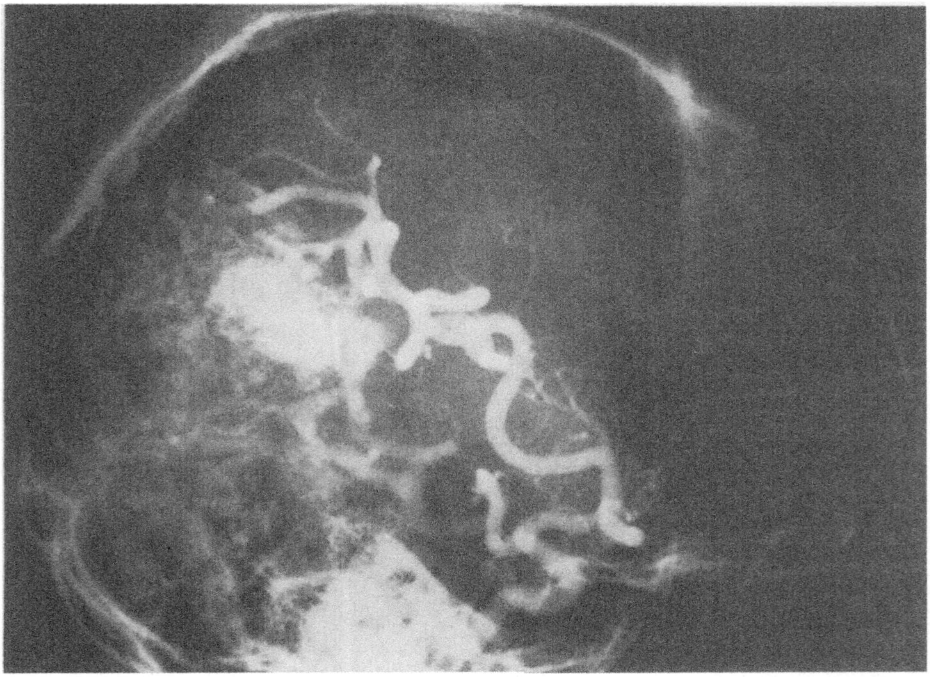

Fig. 3 A. Angiographic findings in man, 24 years, and corresponding to Doppler recordings in Fig. 1, show a large parietal AVM filling from the right middle and posterior cerebral arteries. Left side angiography showed feeder collateral cross-filling into the right MCA via the anterior cerebral artery (not shown)

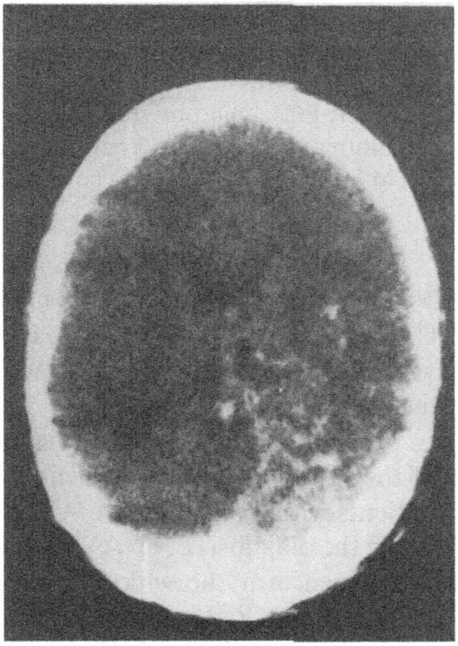

Fig. 3 B. Findings from CT scan with contrast enhancement in this patient shows large right parietal AVM

For the detection of individual AVM feeders sensitivity was 93%. These results confirm the relevance of correlating suspected abnormal findings to reference values from each idividual investigated.

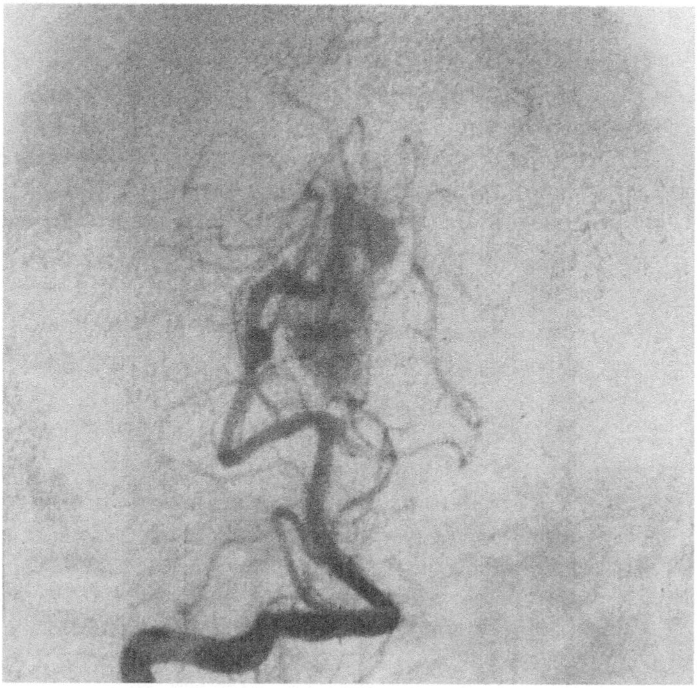

Fig. 3 C. Findings from CT scan within hours after the onset of violent headache in man, aged 42 years. A hematoma of the cerebellar vermis region is seen (arrow). Small area showing increased density after contrast injection (arrowhead) aroused the suspicion of an AVM, which was confirmed by transcranial Doppler (Fig. 2) and by the subsequent angiography (Fig. 3 D)

Extracranial Doppler Investigation

Some patients with cerebral AVM show increased carotid artery (ICA) flow velocities [19]. In the 15 patients with AVM feeders from the carotids, ICA flow velocities ranged from 36 to 85 cm/sec, median: 62 cm/sec on the AVM side and from 28 to 64 cm/sec, median 52 cm/s, on the opposite side. While an increased ICA volume flow was no doubt present in these patients, this effect often seemed to be largely compensated by the associated ICA diameter enlargement. Presuming that ICA flow velocities on opposing sides normally are within $\pm 25\%$ of each other, AVM diagnosis would have to be based on findings of a higher degree of ICA flow velocity assymmetry. In the present series, this criterion was met in 5 patients only, all of whom had a large AVM. Extracranial Doppler investigation seems of limited value in the diagnosis of AVMs. It is not surprising to find that, by virtue of its ability to investigate individual major cerebral arteries selectively, transcranial Doppler is superior for diagnosing and evaluating patients with AVM.

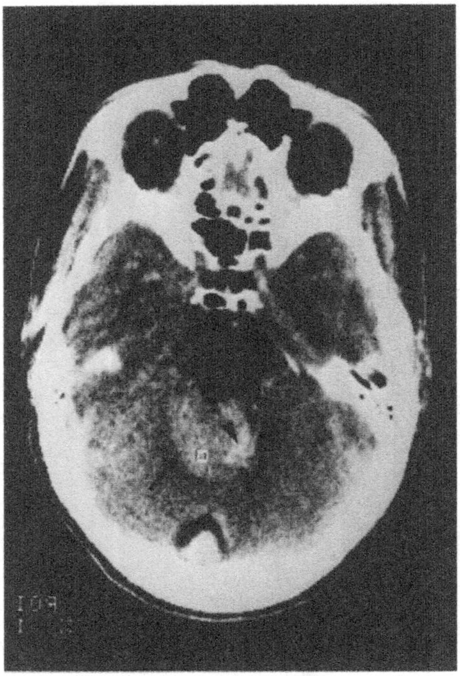

Fig. 3D. Angiographic findings corresponding to CT findings in Fig. 3C and Doppler recordings in Fig. 2. An infratentorial, medium-size AVM is filling from the enlarged right superior cerebellar artery. The posterior cerebral arteries filled from the carotid system bilaterally in this patient (not shown)

Localization of AVMs

The localization of AVMs from transcranial Doppler investigation was obtained by combining findings from individual basal cerebral arteries according to known anatomical principles. Table 1 shows that there was good correlation between the anatomical region occupied by the AVM and the feeder artery having the highest flow velocity. Paramedian AVMs were revealed from the predominant involvement of one, or both, anterior cerebral arteries (ACAs). These findings correspond well with the anatomical knowledge that blood supply to an AVM is through the specific arteries normally supplying this brain region [8]. An ACA feeder collateral cross-filling into the opposite carotid territory was seen in three patients with large hemisphere convexity AVM. The situation was revealed from the retrograde ACA flow on the AVM side, and basically resembles ACA collateral flow in patients with severe carotid artery disease [12].

The number of AVM feeder arteries gave indications as to the anatomical size of the AVM (Table 2). Equally important clinically is that

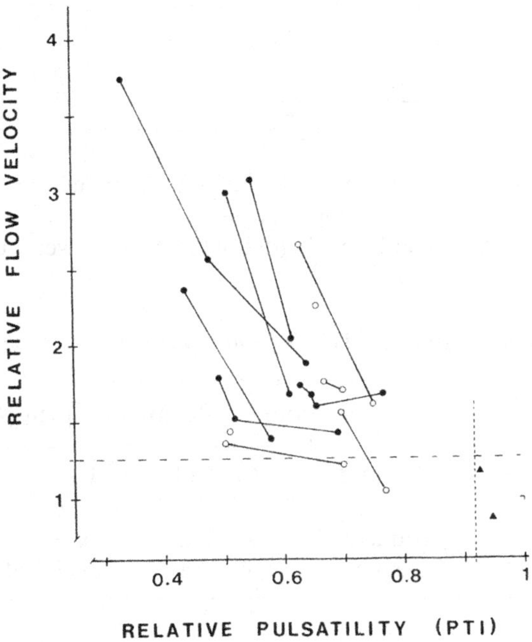

Fig. 4. Findings from AVM feeder arteries normalized against findings from normal remote arteries in individual patients. The point (1.0, 1.0) denotes normal remote arteries. Note the inverse relationship between flow velocity and pulsatility. Findings in patients with large AVMs (dots) were not significantly different from findings in patients with mediumsize AVM's (circles). The limits PTI = 0.92 (punctuated line) and relative flow velocity = 1.25 (broken line) represent two SDs from the means in healthy volunteers. Findings from the feeding arteries to two small AVM's (< 2 cm, triangles) were within this "normal range"

findings of multiple feeders reflect the degree of vascular involvement of an AVM.

Hemodynamic Effects of Arteriovenous Malformations

The vascular resistance in an AVM is low compared to the normal cerebrovascular resistance at normal perfusion pressure and CO_2 levels. This accounts for a very high volume flow and the well-known enlarged diameter of AVM feeder arteries. Flow velocity levels in these channels are characteristically higher than in normal arteries [21].

Table 1. *AVM size and number of feeder arteries*

AVM Size	AVM Feeder Arteries				
	4	3	2	1	Total
Large	1	2	4	—	7
Medium	—	—	4	3	7
Small	—	—	—	2*	2

All AVM feeders angiographically verified as supplying medium and large AVMs were identified by transcranial Doppler.
* Feeder arteries to two small AVMs (diameter < 2 cm) were not demonstrable.

Table 2. *Localization of AVMs from transcranial Doppler findings*

Doppler:	Anatomical Region occupied by AVM			
Feeder artery with highest flow velocity	Frontal or paramedian region	Central or sylvian fissure	Parietal or parieto-occipital	Occipital region
Middle cer. a.	—	2	2	—
Anterior cer. a.	5	—	—	—
Posterior cer. a.	—	—	3	2*
Total (AVMs)	5	2	5	2

* One infratentorial AVM fed by an enlarged superior cerebellar artery gave the impression of representing posterior cerebral artery. Two small AVMs not diagnosed by transcranial Doppler are not included.

The low pulsatile amplitude in AVM feeder arteries is due to several factors. A decreased distal resistance and an increased proximal resistance generally leads to a decrease in pulsatility [4, 12–14, 17]. *Under normal conditions, the pressure spent in conveying bloodflow from the aorta and up to the major brain arteries is of the order of very few mm Hg* [3]. The low pulsatility in AVM feeders is due to the combined effect of the low peripheral resistance in the AVM and the pressure expended along the high velocity inflow channels [20]. We interpret the inverse relationship between flow velocity and pulsatility as illustrating this pressure loss (Fig. 4).

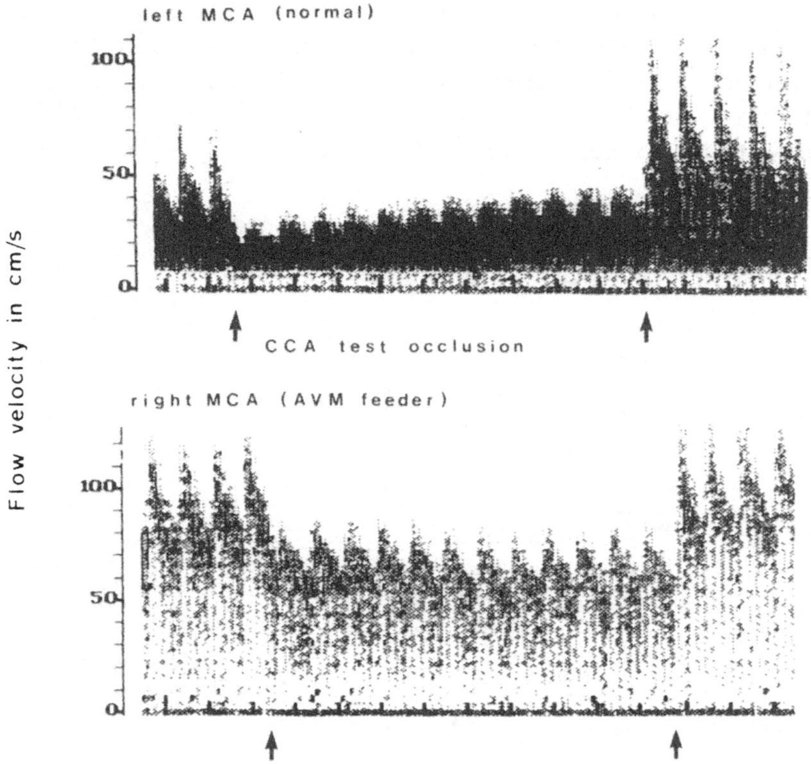

Fig. 5. Test occlusions of the common carotid artery (CCA) in the neck (same patient as in Fig. 1). These MCA recordings were obtained at sampling depth 35 mm to avoid interference from high velocity Willisian collaterals during test occlusions. Flow velocity in the left MCA (normal remote artery) showed a step reduction to 55% of the pre-test level due to the acute drop in MCA perfusion pressure. The autoregulatory response is already visible at three cardiac cycles after the CCA became occluded. Velocity had increased to 75% of the pre-test level after approximately 10 seconds. Following CCA release, MCA flow velocity showed an overshoot to 140% of pre-test level. These findings, and the subsequent velocity regulation back to pretest level, effectfully illustrate the responsiveness of normal cerebrovascular beds. Right MCA (AVM feeder artery) showed a drop to 70% of pretest flow velocity and no secondary flow velocity increase. MCA flow velocity showed a step increase to 105% of pretest level when test occlusion was released, indicating that the net change in the MCA peripheral resistance was very low, owing to the massive influence from the high-flow, nonregulating AVM

Blood Pressure Effects

The MCA inflow pressure was temporarily reduced by means of extracranial CCA test occlusions in 5 patients with AVM supply from the MCA. Each test occlusion lasted about 10 seconds. Sample recordings are shown in Fig. 5. In feeders, as well as in normal remote arteries, flow velocity dropped immediately. This drop showed individual differences which probably illustrate the well-known individual variation in the capacity of Willisian collateral channels. In remote normal arteries, the MCA flow velocity started to increase again almost immediately after the ipsilateral

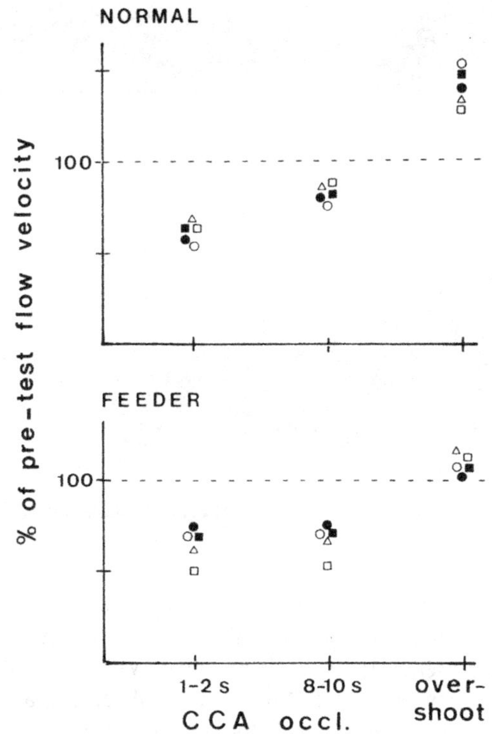

Fig. 6. Middle cerebral artery (MCA) flow velocity responses to ipsilateral common carotid artery (CCA) test occlusion, show a secondary MCA flow velocity increase during test occlusion and a post-occlusion overshoot indicating autoregulation of remote normal brain vasculature (upper). The response in AVM feeders seemed more pressure-passive (lower). Different symbols denote different patients

CCA was occluded, see Fig. 6. This reflects the rapid onset of the autoregulatory response to the reduction in MCA inflow pressure. The secondary increase was less pronounced, or not discernible at all, in AVM feeders. Following the release of test occlusion, when MCA inflow pressure was restored, flow velocity in remote normal arteries transiently exceeded pre-test levels, owing to autoregulated vasculature distal to the recording site. The AVM feeder arteries showed only modest overshoot, further indicating that that flow in these feeders was predominately non-regulated.

The nutrient branches which arise from AVM feeder arteries are beyond reach with the present state of transcranial Doppler instrumentation. However, observations during common carotid artery (CCA) test occlusions in one patient with a frontal midline AVM supplied from the left ACA (Fig. 7), demonstrated some hemodynamic effects which probably are representative of such flow conditions. During the test occlusion of the left CCA in the neck, left MCA flow velocity dropped to 25% of pre-test level and showed no secondary increase (Fig. 8). After eight seconds, the patient reported numbness in the right arm and the right side of the face, indicating impending ischemia in the left MCA territory. Test occlusion was immediately released and was followed by a MCA flow velocity overshoot to 160% of pre-test level, indicating that a powerful vasodilator response had in fact been operative. Due to the low-resistance AVM, antegrade flow persisted in the left ACA, and flow velocity in the left PCA increased from 46 to 180 cm/sec during test occlusion. Despite autoregulation, MCA flow did not increase during test occlusion because the effect from the decreasing peripheral resistance was nullified by concomitantly increasing proximal resistance due to the high velocity collateral inflow.

Right side CCA test occlusion caused MCA velocity drop to 50% of pre-test level. The effect of autoregulation was evidenced from the secondary MCA flow velocity increase which began within one or two heartbeats after test occlusion was established, and from the postocclusive overshoot to 120% of pretest level. Flow velocity in the right PCA increased from 48 to 86 cm/sec during test occlusion.

Following excision of the AVM, the hemodynamic responses to CCA test occlusion were nearly symmetrical, closely resembling those seen on the right side preoperatively, and CCA test occlusion provoked no symptoms.

CO_2 Effects

By acting on the cerebrovascular resistance at the arteriolar level, the arterial CO_2 exerts powerful influence upon blood flow through normal brain [10]. Cerebral blood flow decreases by from 2 to 6% (mean value about 4%) per mm Hg arterial CO_2 reduction [9, 23]. Angiographical observations further indicate that the caliber of large cerebral arteries does not change within the CO_2 range of 25 to 57 mm Hg [7]. Investigating middle cerebral artery flow velocity in healthy volunteers, Markwalder *et al.* demonstrated a vascular reactivity of $3.4 \pm 0.4\%$ per mm Hg (mean and SD) [17]. This is remarkably close to the values for vascular reactivity determined from cerebral blood flow measurements. Acute changes in flow velocity can thus be considered as reflecting actual volume flow variations.

We have studied vascular reactivity in remote normal arteries and feeders in patients with AVM [16]. Using Doppler, the vascular reactivity is defined as the percentage flow velocity change divided by the P_aCO_2 (end

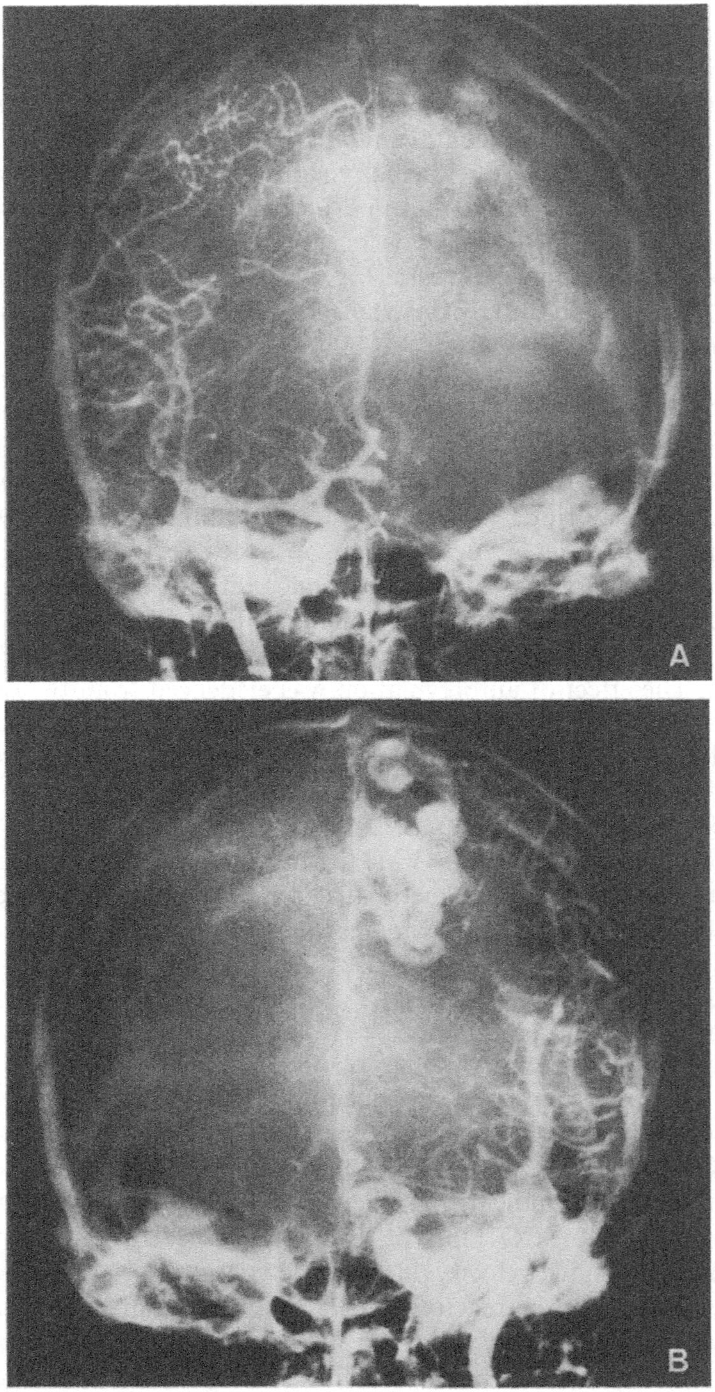

Fig. 7. Findings from angiography and CT in woman, 32 years. The medium-size, left paramedian AVM was fed from the left anterior cerebral artery (ACA). Note enlargement of left ACA when compared to right ACA. CT scanning with contrast enhancement was suggestive of an AVM. The lesion could not be seen from nonenhanced scans

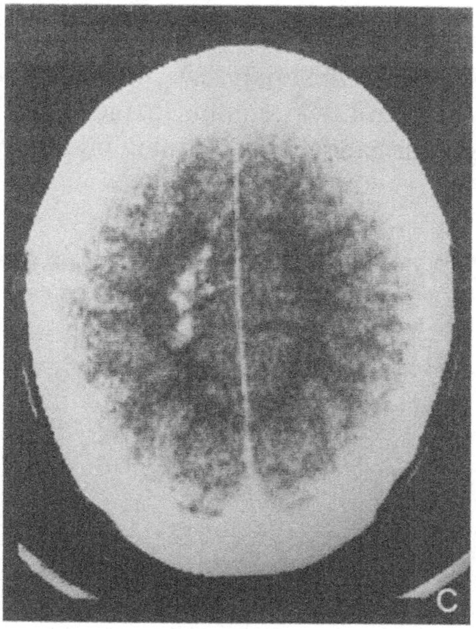

Fig. 7 C

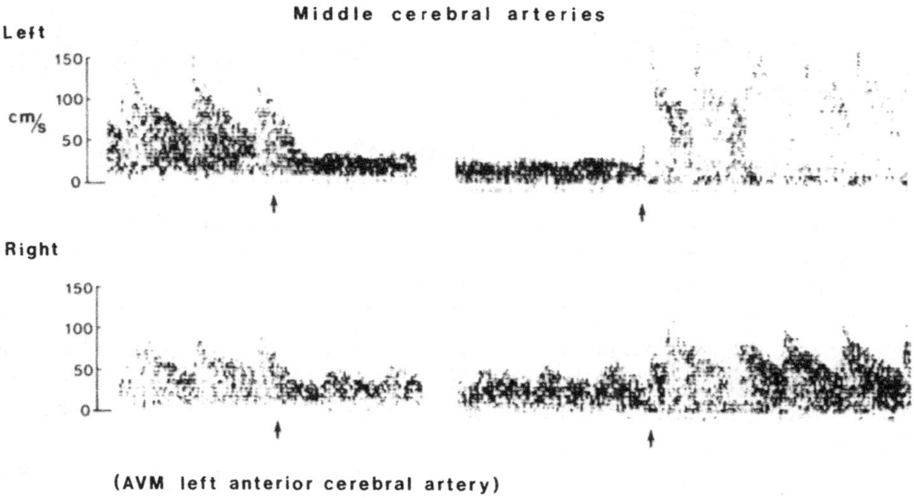

Fig. 8. Test occlusions of the common carotid arteries. Transcranial Doppler recordings obtained from the left (upper) and right (lower) middle cerebral arteries (MCAs). Following ipsilateral test occlusion (between arrows) right MCA flow velocity dropped to 50% of pretest level followed by a secondary velocity increase to 76% of pretest level. Note rapid onset of autoregulation. When test occlusion was released after 10 seconds, MCA flow velocity showed an overshoot to 128% of the pretest value. Left side test occlusion caused a MCA flow velocity drop to 24% of pretest level, which remained unchanged during the occlusion period. After 8 seconds the patient reported numbness of the right face and arm. Following release of test occlusion MCA velocities increased to 160% of pretest level, which indicates that autoregulation in fact had taken place, but its effect on flow had been nullified by increased impedance to flow through collateral channels supplying the AVM at the same time, see Fig. 5

tidal CO_2 measured by infrared analyzer). Normal remote arteries showed vascular reactivity of 2.3 to 4.0% per mm Hg, median: 3.1%, demonstrating a CO_2-dependency characteristic of normal brain flow. Feeder arteries

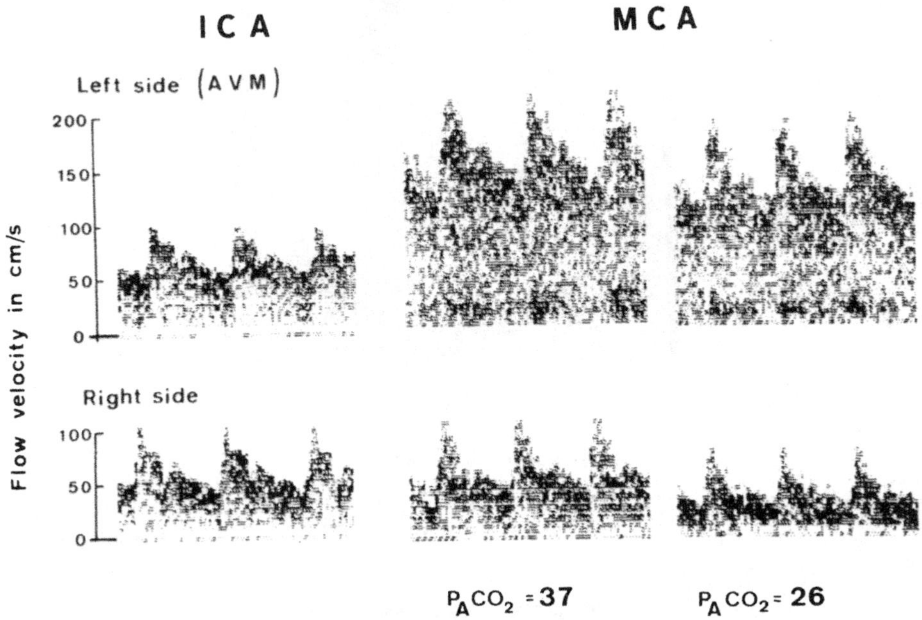

Fig. 9. Doppler recordings before and during hyperventilation test in woman, 18 years (large AVM in the left Sylvian fissure region, see Fig. 10). Flow velocity levels in the distal extracranial internal carotid arteries were nearly symmetrical. The effect from increased volume flow in the left ICA seemed to be off-set by the enlarged ICA diameter and by the fact that the right ICA perfused the distal anterior cerebral arteries bilaterally. Hyperventilation test (far right) reduced P_aCO_2 from 37 to 26 mm Hg. Flow velocity in left MCA (AVM feeder) was reduced from 166 to 142 cm/sec (16% reduction), corresponding to 1.5%/mm Hg. This low vascular reactivity reflects a reduced coupling between CO_2 and flow in this AVM feeder artery. When viewed in context with angiography (Fig. 10) it seems probable that the vascular reactivity reflects the ratio of AVM flow to nutrient flow in feeder arteries. In the remote normal right MCA, flow velocity declined from 70 to 44 cm/sec (37% reduction). Calculated vascular reactivity: 3.4%/mm Hg, is within normal limits

showed vascular reactivity from about zero to 2.4%per mm Hg, significantly lower than in normal remote arteries. Hyperventilation tests thus enhance the value of transcranial Doppler investigation, see Figs. 9, 10, and 11.

Differential Diagnosis

Cerebral Vasospasm

Flow velocities in slightly and moderatly vasospastic cerebral arteries after aneurysmal subarachnoid hemorrhage [1] are often of the same magnitude as those seen in AVM feeder arteries. It is therefore diagnostically important

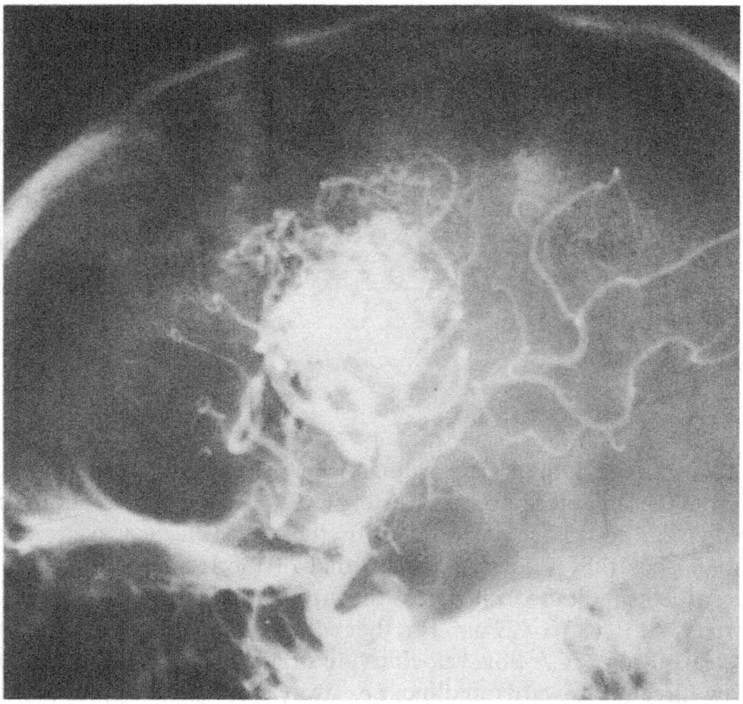

Fig. 10. Left carotid angiography showing a large AVM in the left Sylvian fissure region. Doppler recordings from this patient are shown in Fig. 9

to discriminate between high flow velocities signalling vasospasm and the increased velocity levels which are due to high volume flow in feeders. Hyperventilation tests can be used to demonstrate reduced CO_2 -dependency in AVM feeders. By constrast, the CO_2 -dependency of cerebral flow is near normal in patients with slight or moderate vasospasm [28].

Intracranial Artery Stenosis

Atheromatous arterial stenoses are usually quite short and have an abrupt outlet tract. From transcranial Doppler investigation, these lesions are recognized as representing localized vessel segments where high flow velocities prevail [15]. Doppler signals recorded from these sites therefore also contain low frequency, high intensity components. Poststenotic disturbed flow and wall flutter give rise to these "gruffy" Doppler audio

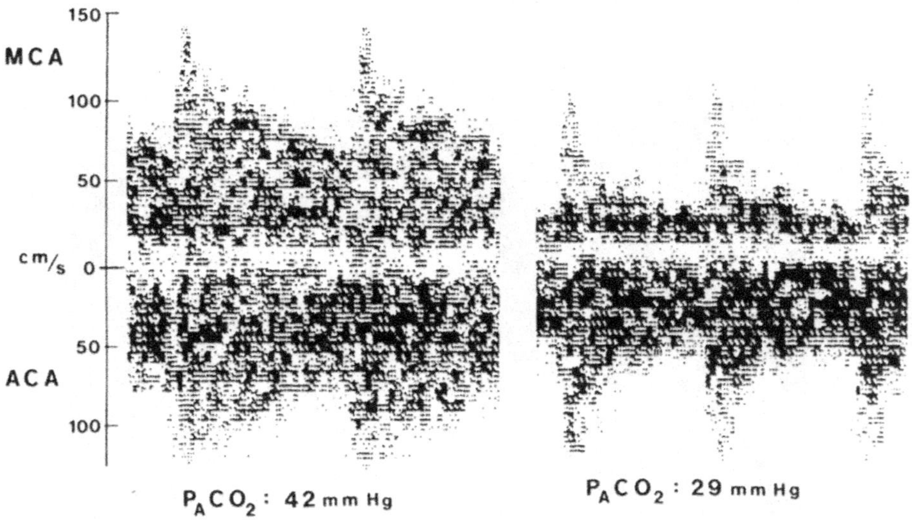

Fig. 11. Transcranial Doppler recording from patient with medium-size AVM supplied from the left anterior cerebral artery (ACA). Angiography shown in Fig. 5. Hyperventilation test is used to identify the AVM feeder artery which, at normocapnia, has flow velocity equal to that of the left middle cerebral artery (MCA) recorded simultaneously across the intracranial bifurcation of the internal carotid artery. At P_ACO_2 of 29 mm Hg, the reduced vascular reactivity in the AVM feeder is clearly seen. ACA flow velocities are shown below the zero line to denote flow direction towards midline, *i.e.*, away from the Doppler probe

signals which are typically different from the smooth character of Doppler signals recorded from normal intracranial arteries or from AVM feeders.

Willisian Collaterals

Extracranial carotid artery disease is reliably identified using extracranial Doppler techniques [11]. The differentiation between AVM feeders and high velocity collaterals in the circle of Willis nevertheless deserves comment. In patients with an AVM supplied purely from one or more of the vessels in the circle of Willis, *i.e.*, the proximal anterior or posterior cerebral arteries, the high flow velocity patterns may resemble those seen when these vessels provide collateral flow to the middle cerebral artery [12]. The transcranial Doppler technique also provides information to identify the inflow source to individual vessels. This is accomplished using test occlusions of the common carotid artery which aid the identification of the vessel investigated [12]. True collateral flow across the circle of Willis prevails in some patients with AVM. Such feeder collaterals are recognized from the high flow velocity pattern also present in the recipient middle cerebral artery.

Although not represented in the present series, very large AVMs involving all major basal cerebral arteries do occur. A remote normal artery may then not be available for reference. We would, however, expect that this extreme condition could be revealed from conspiciously high flow velocities and low PI values in all basal cerebral arteries and from the low vasomotor reactivity during hyperventilation tests.

Conclusions and Clinical Implications

Transcranial Doppler investigations provide two basically different types of diagnostic information which permit the identification of individual cerebral arteries and hence, the diagnosis and anatomical localization of an AVM: the high flow velocity and the low PI seen in recordings from AVM feeder arteries. Transcranial Doppler investigation also permits reliable identification of individual basal cerebral arteries [12]. The localization of an AVM can therefore be obtained in accordance with the anatomical knowledge that blood supply to an AVM is through the arteries normally supplying the brain region involved. Hyperventilation tests further enhance diagnostic capability.

In many patients with AVM a noninvasive diagnosis is possible using transcranial Doppler alone. In the present series, transcranial Doppler permitted a correct diagnosis in 87% of the patients and in 93% of angiographically verified AVM feeder arteries. It should, however, be realized that these figures mainly reflect the number of small AVMs in our series. Nevertheless, postoperative normal pressure breakthough due to deficient autoregulation in brain vasculature adjacent to an AVM seems to occur after exclusion of high-flow AVMs only [20, 22, 24, 25]. These lesions, which are of particular concern to the operating surgeon, can be readily evaluated with transcranial Doppler investigation.

Patients with AVMs are increasingly accepted for surgical treatment, even at the risk of some permanent neurologic deficit following the exclusion of an AVM [22, 27]. In clinical practice, we have found transcranial Doppler to be a useful addition to CT scanning for primary diagnosis and for the planning of angiography. Adequate angiographic evaluation of patients considered for surgical treatment remains indispensible; however, the surgeons judgement in the individual patient also comprises an estimation of the vascular complexity of an AVM [18, 20, 22]. To this end, transcranial Doppler provides means to investigate and to assess the individual hemodynamic state. This type of information appears not to be obtainable by other investigation techniques.

Transcranial Doppler furthermore seems clinically interesting as a complement to angiography in patients in whom treatment by means of high focus radiation or flow-carried emboli is selected [6, 26], and offers the prospect of reducing the number of X-ray exposures required in follow-up of these patients.

Acknowledgement

This work was supported by Norwegian Council on Cardiovascular Diseases.

References

1. Aaslid R, Huber P, Nornes H (1984) Evaluation of cerebrovascular spasm with transcranial Doppler ultrasound. J Neurosurg 60: 37–41
2. Aaslid R, Markwalder T-M, Nornes H (1982) Noninvasive transcranial Doppler ultrasound recording of flow velocity in basal cerebral arteries. J Neurosurg 57: 769–774
3. Bakay L, Sweet WH (1952) Cervical and intracranial intraarterial pressures with and without vascular occlusions. Surg Gynecol Obstet 95: 67–72
4. Evans DH, Barrie WW, Asher MJ, *et al.* (1980) The relationship between ultrasonic pulsatility index and proximal arterial stenosis in a canine model. Circ Res 46: 470–475
5. Gosling RG, King DH (1974) Arterial assessment by Doppler shift ultrasound. Proc R Soc Med 67: 447–449
6. Hilal SK (1984) Endovascular treatment of arteriovenous malformations of the central nervous system. In: Wilson CB, Stein BM (eds): Inracranial arteriovenous malformations. Williams and Wilkins, Baltimore, pp 259–273
7. Huber P, Handa J (1967) Effect of contrast material, hypercapnia, hyperventilation, hypertonic glucose and paparverine on the diameter of the cerebral arteries—angiographic determination in man. Invest Radiol 2: 17–32
8. Kaplan HA, Aronson SM, Bowder EJ (1961) Vascular malformations of the brain. An anatomical study. J Neurosurg 18: 630–635
9. Kety SS, Schmidt CF (1948) The effects of altered tensions of carbon dioxide and oxygen on cerebral blood flow and cerebral oxygen consumption of normal young men. J Clin Invest 27: 484–492
10. Lassen NA (1974) Control of cerebral circulation in health and disease. Circ Res 34: 749–760
11. Lindegaard K-F, Bakke SJ, Grip A, *et al* (1984) Pulsed Doppler techniques for measuring instantaneous maximum and mean flow velocities in carotid arteries. Ultrasound Med Biol 10: 419–426

12. Lindegaard K-F, Bakke SJ, Grolimund P, *et al* (1985) Carotid artery disease: Assessment of intracranial hemodynamic pattern by noninvasive transcranial Doppler ultrasound. J Neurosurg 63: 890–898
13. Lindegaard K-F, Grip A, Nornes H (1980) Precerebral haemodynamics in brain tamponade. Part 1: Clinical studies on blood flow velocity. Neurochirurgia (Stuttg) 23: 133–142
14. Lindegaard K-F, Grip A, Nornes H (1980) Precerebral hemodynamics in brain tamponade. Part 2: Experimental studies. Neurochirurgia (Stuttg) 23: 187–196
15. Lindegaard K-F, Bakke SJ, Aaslid R, *et al* (1986) Doppler diagnosis of intracranial artery occlusive disorders. J Neurol Neurosurg Psychiat 47: 510–518
16. Lindegaard K-F, Grolimund P, Aaslid R *et al* (1986) Evaluation of cerebral arteriovenous malformations using transcranial Doppler ultrasound. J Neurosurg 65 (in press)
17. Markwalder T-M, Grolimund P, Seiler RW, *et al* (1984) Dependency of blood flow velocity in the middle cerebral artery on end tidal carbon dioxide partial pressure. A transcranial Doppler study. J Cereb Blood Flow Metab 4: 368–372
18. Mullan S, Brown FD, Patronas NJ (1979) Hyperemic and ischemic problems of surgical treatment of arteriovenous malformations. J Neurosurg 51: 757–764
19. Nies JM (1976) The hemodynamic effect of an intracranial arteriovenous anomaly. Clin Neurol Neurosurg 79: 29–45
20. Nornes H, Grip A (1980) Hemodynamic aspects of cerebral arteriovenous malformations. J Neurosurg 53: 456–464
21. Nornes H, Grip A, Wikeby P (1979) Intraoperative evaluation of cerebral hemodynamics using directional Doppler technique. Part 1: Arteriovenous malformations. J Neurosurg 50: 145–151
22. Nornes H, Lundar T, Wikeby P (1979) Cerebral arteriovenous malformations; results of microsurgical management. Acta Neurochir (Wien) 50: 243–257
23. Olesen J, Paulson OB, Lassen NA (1971) Regional cerebral blood flow in man determined by the inital slope of the clearance of intra-arterially injected 133Xe. Stroke 2: 519–540
24. Solomon RA, Michelsen WJ (1984) Detective cerebrovascular autoregulation in regions proximal to arteriovenous malformations of the brain: A case report and topic review. Neurosurgery 14: 78–82
25. Spetzler RF, Wilson CB, Weinstein P, *et al* (1978) Normal perfusion pressure break-through theory. Clin Neurosurg 25: 651–672
26. Steiner L (1984) Treatment of arteriovenous malformations by radiosurgery.In: Wilson CB, Stein BM (eds) Intracranial arteriovenous malformations. Williams and Wilkins, Baltimore, pp 259–273
27. Trumpy JH, Eldevik P (1977) Intracranial arteriovenous malformations: Conservative or surgical treatment? Surg Neurol 8: 171–175
28. Voldby B, Enevoldsen EM, Jensen FT (1985) Cerebrovascular reactivity in patients with ruptured intracranial aneurysms. J Neurosurg 62: 59–67

Author's address: Dr. K.-F. Lindegaard, Department of Neurosurgery, Rikshospitalet, N-0027 Oslo 1, Norway.

7. Comparison of Intraoperative and Transcranial Doppler

J. Gilsbach and *A. Harders*

Introduction

The first intraoperative Doppler investigations of intracranial arteries were described in 1979 by Nornes *et al.* They used a 6 and 10 MHz pulsed system in combination with small probes to record Doppler shifts from intracranial vessels. In 1983, Gilsbach reported on the use of a 20 MHz high resolution system which permitted the investigation of vessels as small as 0.1 mm in diameter, using sterilizable microprobes. Since the introduction of transcranial Doppler sonography by Aaslid in 1982, comparisons between the pre- and postoperative transcranial findings and the direct intraoperative recordings of the same vessel in an individual patient have become possible.

The direct comparability of the Doppler findings is, however, to some extent restricted because of the different incident angles, the special conditions of the open and closed skull, and the different Doppler systems including a ten times higher emitting frequency of the intraoperative device.

Material and Method

The intraoperative recordings were performed with a 20 MHz pulsed Doppler system with miniaturized sterilizable probes* (Table 1). The incident angle was adjusted acoustically and under direct vision, so that the Doppler signal was optimized to provide the highest frequencies. This was usually the case with an angle of 50 to 60 degrees. The gate was adjusted to the center stream. The depth of the gate (axial resolution) was usually chosen between 0.4 and 0.7 mm (250 and 450 nsec). The maximum detectable frequencies were 12.5 kHz due to the filter arrangements, not due to the pulse repetition frequency which was 100 kHz. Therefore in cases with high velocities, such as in vasospasm and angiomas, the systolic peaks were

* MF 20 Microvascular Doppler manufactured by Eden Medizinische Elektronik (EME), Ueberlingen, Federal Republic of Germany.

Table 1. *Technical data of the Doppler device*

20 MHz pulsed ultrasonic Doppler velocimeter	
Transmitted frequency	20 mHz
Pulse durations	250, 450, 850 nsec
Axial resolution	0.4, 0.7, 1.3 mm
Lateral resolutions	0.5, 1.1 mm
Pulse repetition frequencies	25, 50, 100 kHz
Measuring depth	maximum 15 mm
Adjustable in steps of 0.1 mm	
Maximum detectable Doppler shift	12.5 kHz
Minimum detectable Doppler shift	0.1 kHz

cut. The evaluation of the main frequencies with the built-in zero crossing system and recorder was abandoned in favor of the interpretation of the complete spectrum and the maximum velocity envelope by a real time frequency analyzer (Angioscan). Since this initial study, we now use an instrument with a built-in FFT spectrum analyzer and an improved filtering system which allows measurement of velocities of up to 22 kHz with autoclavalable probes from 1 mm in diameter (Figs. 1 and 2)*.

Transcranial recordings were originally performed with an Aaslid prototype 2 MHz pulsed Doppler, and for the last six months of the study with a TC 2–64 Transcranial Doppler* with an antialiasing FFT system which enabled the measurement of frequencies up to 10 kHz.

Results

Normal Cases

In cases of small basal tumors and optic nerve tumors, normal vessels could be recorded under open operative conditions. The velocities in the middle cerebral and internal carotid artery were nearly the same, whereas the velocities in the horizontal part of the anterior cerebral arteries were moderately slower. Resistance indices were between 0.2 and 0.7. These findings were consistant with those found transcranially, which also showed slower velocities in the anterior cerebral artery. The comparison of the absolute velocities, with respect to an angle of sixty degrees and a ten times

* Eden Medizinische Elektronik (EME), Ueberlingen, Federal Republic of Germany.

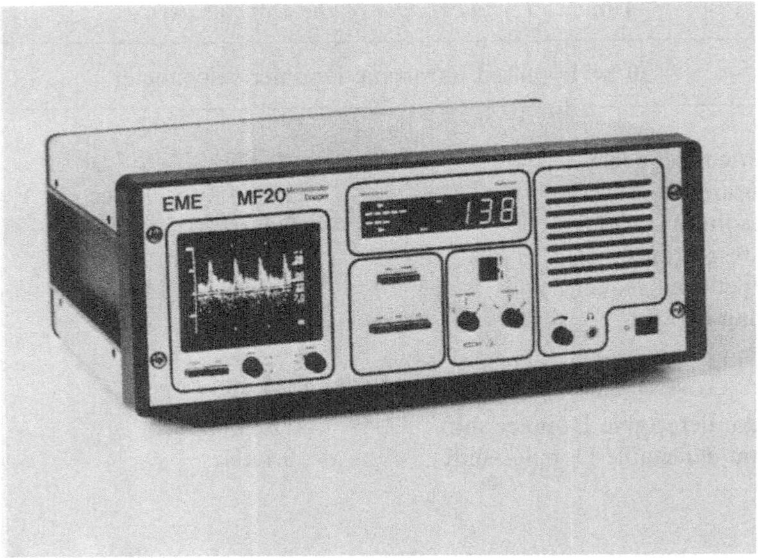

Fig. 1. The present MF 20 Microvascular Doppler device with built-in FFT spectrum analyzer (EME, Ueberlingen)

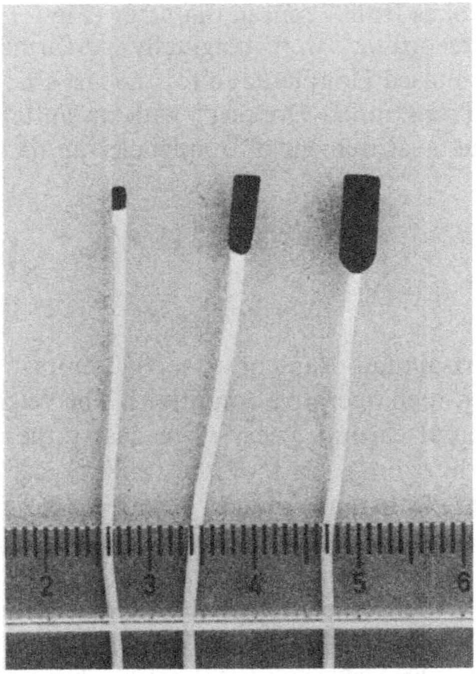

Fig. 2. The autoclavable microprobes for intraoperative use

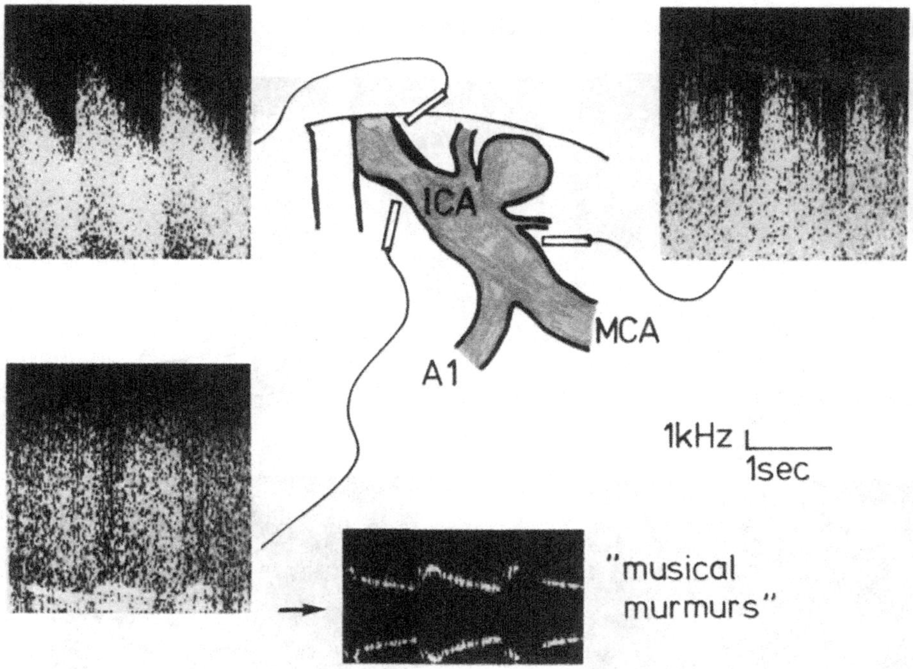

Fig. 3 a. Posterior communicating artery aneurysm with moderate stenosis (spasm?) of the proximal intracranial carotid artery. The intraoperative Doppler reveals a moderate acceleration but also "musical murmurs" as a sign of wall vibrations

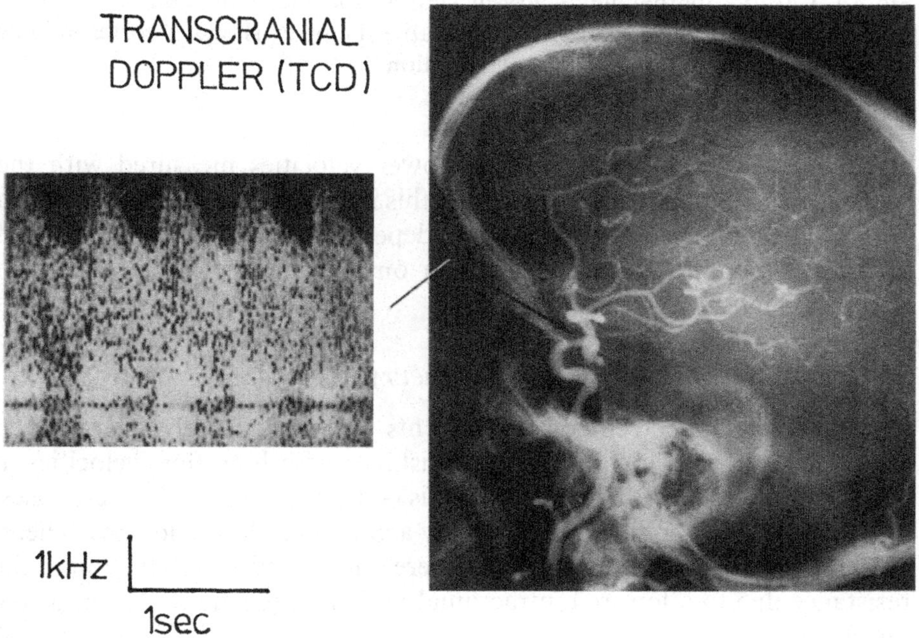

Fig. 3 b. The transcranial findings of the same patient (Fig. 3 a) show a local acceleration in the internal carotid artery with a signal similar to the cry of a seagull

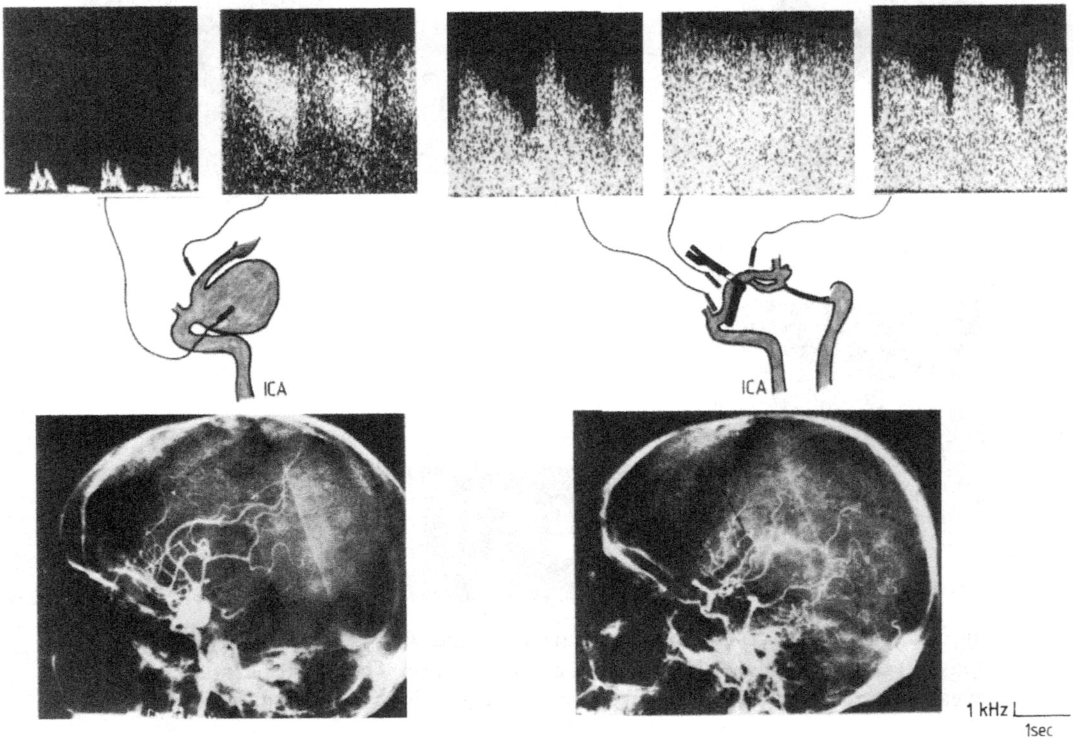

Fig. 4a. Carotid-ophthalmic aneurysm with a moderate reduction of the vessel caliber due to a tight clip. The intraoperative Doppler shows a corresponding acceleration

higher emitting frequency, revealed lower velocities measured with the microvascular Doppler. The reason for this intraoperative underestimation of the velocities is not clear. Perhaps it depends on the special condition of the open skull, differences in $paCO_2$ or on the filter arrangements which affect the higher frequencies.

Cerebral Aneurysms

In more than 50 percent of the patients operated acutely on ruptured aneurysms, signs of low peripheral resistance with high flow velocities in nearly all segments of the circle of Willis could be detected. In these cases, angiography showed normal or slightly accelerated flow velocities. Therefore, the intraoperative accelerations were interpreted as a reduction of the resistance due to a lowered intracranial pressure after trephination or the release of CSF.

The intraoperative hyperemia was more marked in patients with severe subarachnoid bleedings, and these patients developed more postoperative

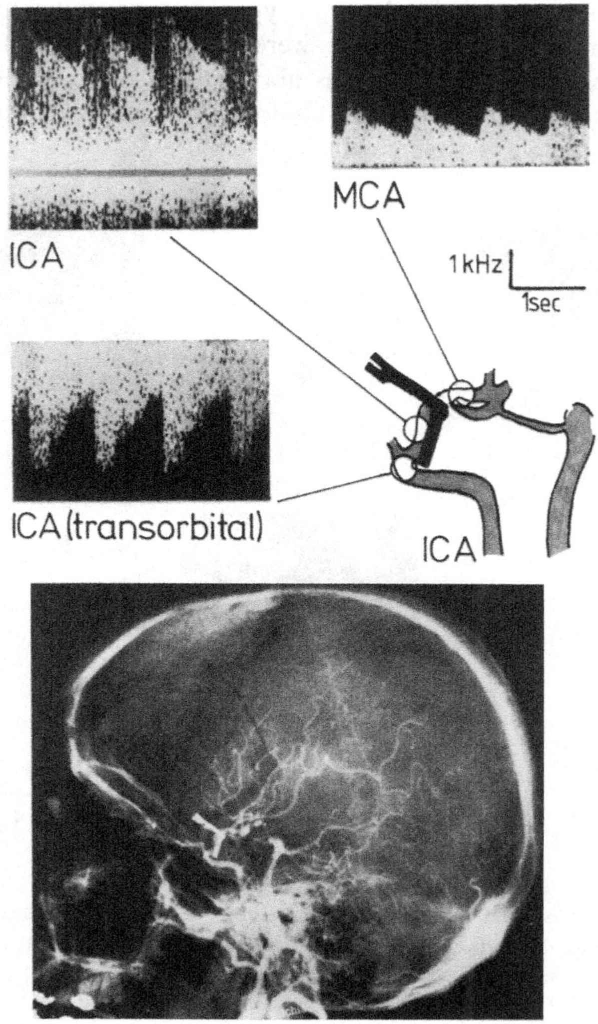

Fig. 4 b. A similar moderate acceleration of the internal carotid artery could also be detected transcranially with the TCD

spasms, with an earlier and more rapid increase of the velocities detected with the transcranial system.

The most significant flow disturbances in delayed aneurysm surgery were vasospasms. In 74 percent of the patients operated upon after the 4th day following the bleeding, we found varying degrees of accelerations due to lumen narrowing. These findings correlated well with the transcranial recordings (Figs. 3 a and b, 4 a and b, 5 a and b). Musical murmurs could also be found intraoperatively (Fig. 3). While the transcranial measurements—at least with the prototype—were restricted by the aliasing effect, the intraoperative recordings were influenced by the inability of the earlier device to detect frequencies above 12.5 kHz. Therefore the flow patterns from the different systems could not be compared with each other in cases of severe vasospasms with high velocities.

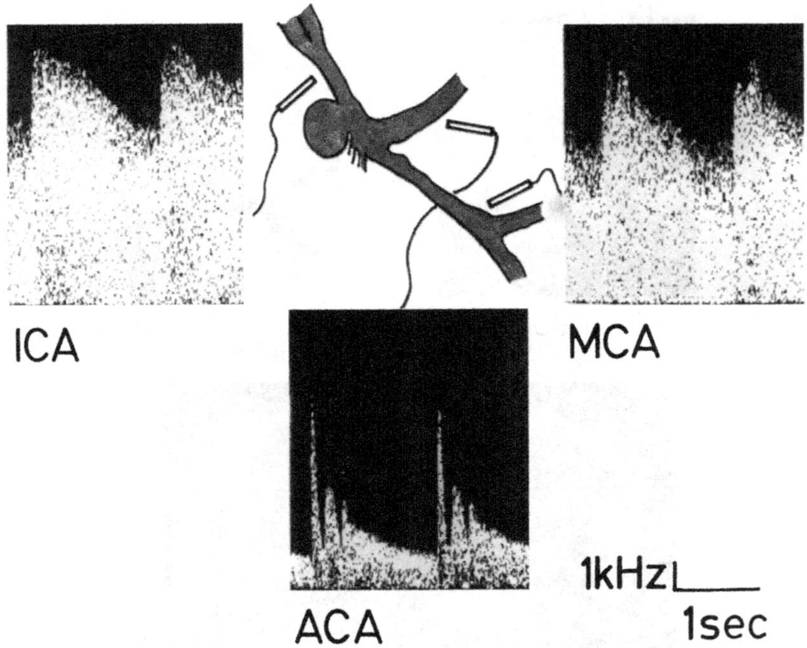

Fig. 5 a

Figs. 5 a and b. Posterior communicating artery aneurysm with marked spasms of the internal carotid and middle cerebral artery both intraoperatively and transcranially

Maximal vasospasms were normally not recorded intraoperatively because the operation was postponed when severe vasospasms were diagnosed from the transcranial Doppler recordings. In the patients operated upon with moderate vasospasms, the intraoperative flow pattern corresponded to those obtained transcranially.

The intraoperative patency control with the high resolution Doppler system could be controlled and repeated transcranially (Figs. 4 a and b). In the early postoperative phase we saw no discrepancies.

Extracranial-intracranial Bypass

The intraoperative recordings of the recipient vessel revealed varying degrees of pathologically low flow velocities, with damped pulse curves

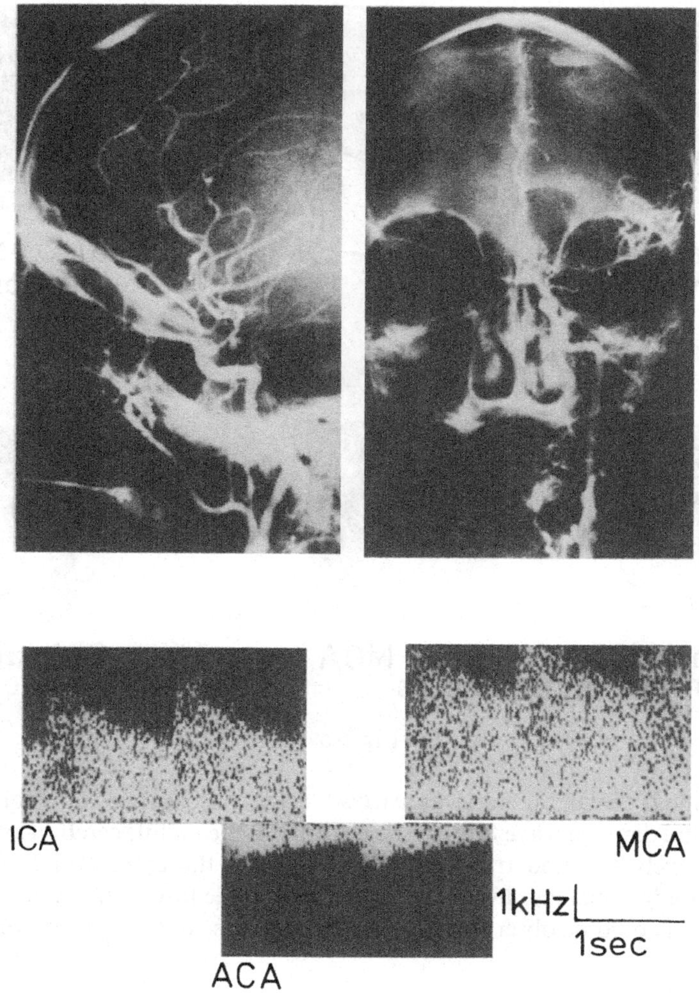

Fig. 5 b

depending on the occluded or stenosed vessels (Fig. 6 a). The same flow pattern could also be recorded transcranially in the region of the middle cerebral artery branches (Fig. 6 b). In patients with only one occluded carotid artery and TIA, the incidence of normal or nearly normal flow pattern of the recipient artery was 50 percent.

In 97 percent of all patients, a bilateral flow distribution was present in the recipient artery after the anastomosis, with high inward flow velocities mainly to the Sylvian fissure. In these cases, the velocities in the donor artery increased, and the resistance index decreased, so that a change from the external to the internal type could be observed. The transcranial Doppler findings also revealed retrograde flow of a similar percentage in the territory

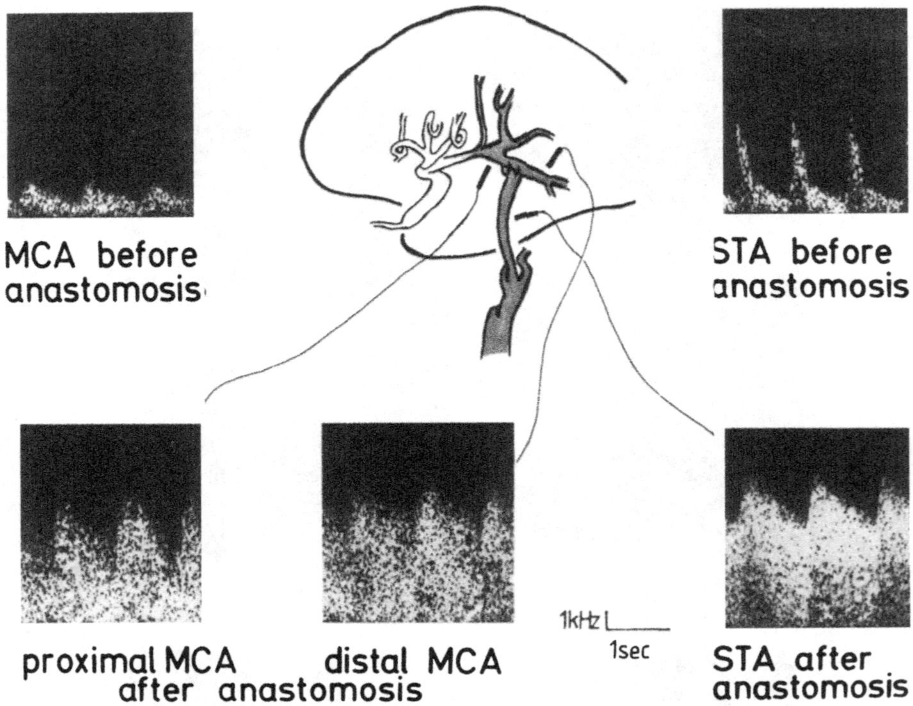

Fig. 6a

Figs. 6a and b. Bilateral cervical carotid artery occlusion. Slow blood flow velocities and damped wave form in the territory of the middle cerebral artery, both intraoperatively *(a)* and transcranially *(b)*. After the extracranial-intracranial bypass procedure increased velocities and a retrograde flow in the recipient middle cerebral area could be observed, as well as an increase of flow in the donor artery

of the middle cerebral artery vessels. Sometimes it reversed to its original orthograde direction on compression of the donor artery (Fig. 6b). These findings corresponded well to the intraoperative recorded retrograde flow towards the Sylvian fissure.

The detection of the increased flow velocity in the distal part of the anastomosis was not possible transcranially in all cases, so that a high orthograde flow velocity could be observed only in some cases.

In patients in which the patency of the anastomosis was demonstrated intraoperatively with the high frequency Doppler, the early postoperative transcranial Doppler control also showed a functioning anastomosis.

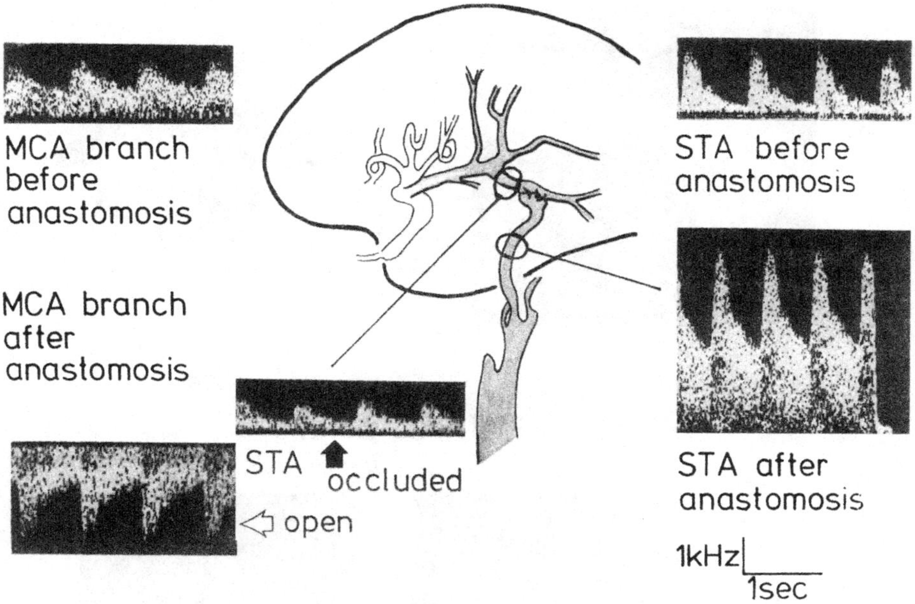

Fig. 6 b

Angioma

Both intraoperatively and transcranially, the Doppler sonographic signs of a flow with a low resistance could be detected in angioma feeding vessels (Figs. 7 a and b). After exclusion of the fistulas, the signs of high peripheral resistance could be detected intraoperatively in vessels which fed both angioma and normal brain. This could be also observed transcranially in the postoperative course.

Conclusion

Comparison between the intraoperative, visually controlled Doppler findings and the transcranial examinations indicate that a pathological flow patterns in transcranial Doppler sonography can be identified in the individual vessel with a high degree of reliability. Changes in the flow pattern due to the operation should be further investigated with simultaneous intraoperative and transcranial recordings.

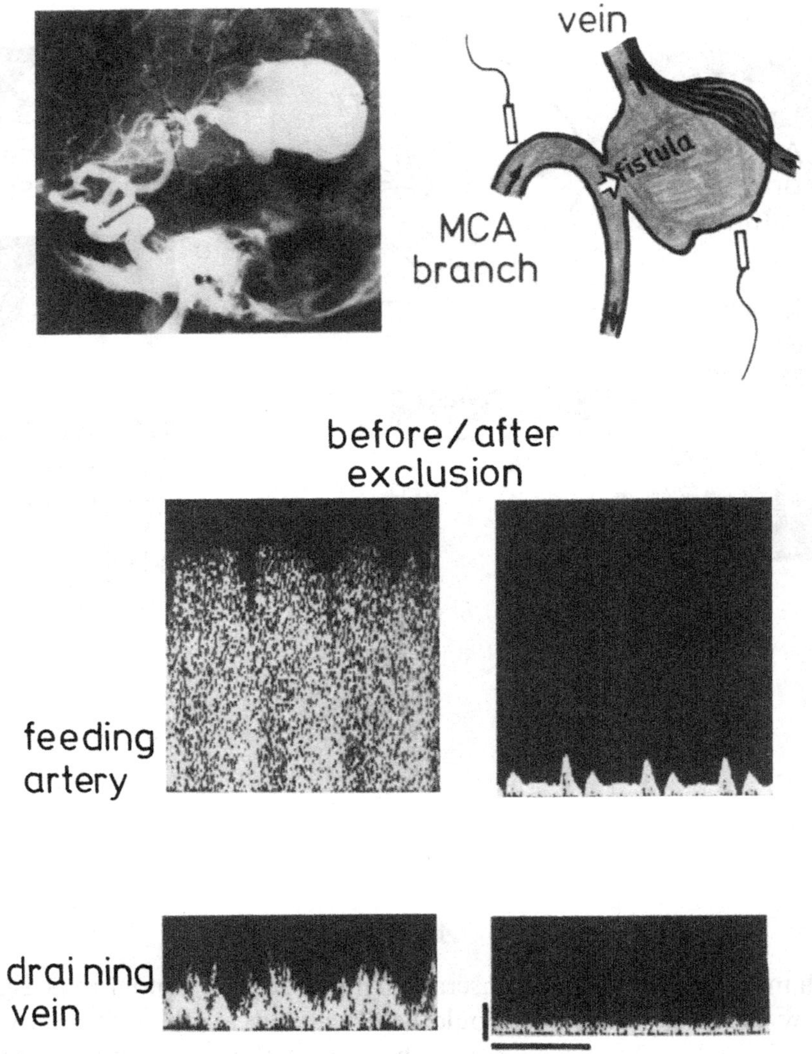

Fig. 7 a

Figs. 7 a and b. Arteriovenous fistula fed by a branch of the middle cerebral artery with high flow velocities and a high enddiastolic flow as a sign of a reduced peripheral resistance. After exclusion of the angioma, signs of an increased resistance in the former angioma feeding artery could be observed

ARTERIO-VENOUS FISTULA AND TRANSCRANIAL DOPPLER

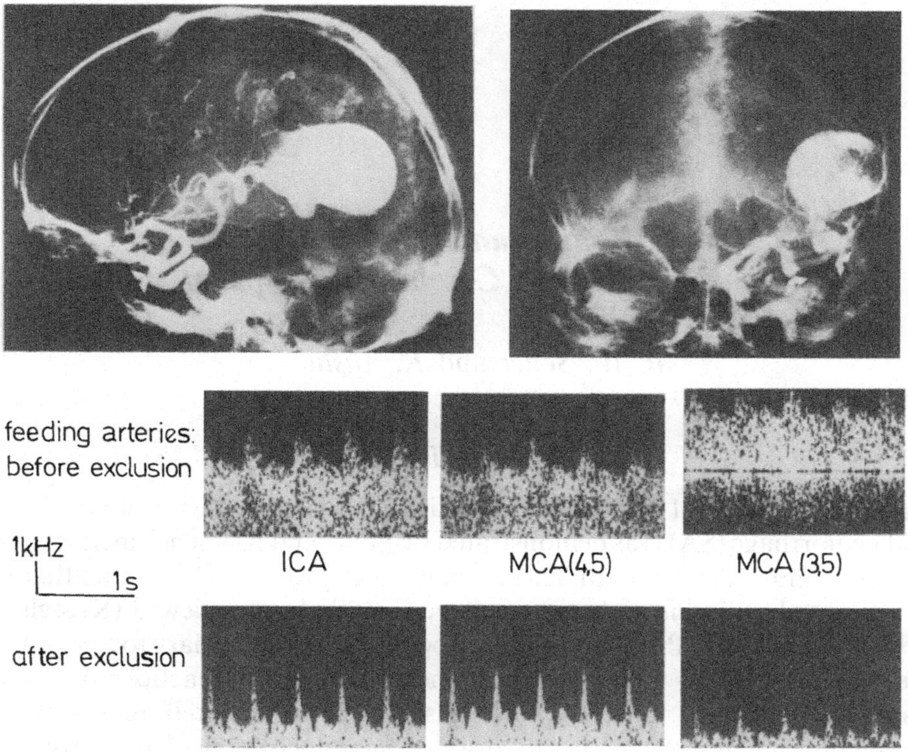

References

Aaslid R, Markwalder T-M, Nornes H (1982) Noninvasive transcranial Doppler ultrasound recording of flow velocity in basal cerebral arteries. J Neurosurg 57: 769–774

Gilsbach JM (1983) Intraoperative Doppler sonography in neurosurgery. Springer, Wien New York

Nornes H, Grip A, Wickeby P (1979) Intraoperative evaluation of cerebral hemodynamics using directional Doppler technique. Part 1, arteriovenous malformations. J Neurosurg 50: 145–151

Nornes H, Grip A, Wickeby P (1979) Intraoperative evaluation of cerebral hemodynamics using directional Doppler technique. Part 2, saccular aneurysms. J Neurosurg 50: 570–577

Nornes H, Grip A (1980) Hemodynamic aspects of cerebral arteriovenous malformations. J Neurosurg 53: 456–464

Author's address: Prof. Dr. J. Gilsbach, Neurochirurgische Universitätsklinik, Hugstetter Strasse 55, D-7800 Freiburg i. Br., Federal Republic of Germany.

8. Transcranial Doppler for Evaluation of Cerebral Vasospasm

R. W. Seiler and *R. Aaslid*

Introduction

Spasm of the cerebral arteries is a complication associated with subarachnoid hemorrhage (SAH) as demonstrated by Ecker and Riemenschneider in 1951. It is most likely a multifactorial multistage process. The factors that may be involved in his pathogenesis have recently been reviewed (Kassell 1985, Wellum 1985). Probably initial vasoconstriction secondary to vasoactive substances leads to degeneration and inflammatory reactions of the vessel wall, so that in severe vasospasm (VSP) the initial functional contraction finally results in an organic vasculopathy with structural changes of the wall and narrowing of the lumen of the blood vessels (Hughes 1978).

The hemodynamic effect of VSP is similar to that of a stenosis, both producing an increase in blood flow velocity and a loss of pressure through the narrow segment (Blaumanis 1979). Cerebral blood flow (CBF) will be reduced when autoregulation in the distal vascular bed has been exhausted and is unable to compensate for the increased resistance of the spastic segment. Because of sufficient collateral circulation and the effectiveness of cerebral autoregulation, the majority of patients with SAH have no critical reduction of CBF, although their cerebral arteries may exhibit some degree of VSP in angiography. CBF is reduced to a critical level only when the compensatory capacity of the vasoregulatory mechanism has been exhausted, leading to ischemia or infarction, so that cerebral VSP becomes clinically symptomatic. In patients with aneurysmal SAH who reach neurosurgical centers, infarction from VSP is still the leading cause of death and disability.

For the evaluation of the efficacy of any treatment and the timing of operation, the development and resolution of the arterial narrowing should be monitored. Angiography, the standard method of assessing cerebral

VSP, is an invasive procedure that cannot be repeated at frequent intervals. With the transcranial ultrasonic Doppler technique it is possible to record the increased velocity in the spastic arterial segment. Because the velocity of blood flow is inversely related to the lumen area (Blaumanis 1979), the arterial narrowing can be evaluated by this method. Since transcranial Doppler ultrasound (TCD) is noninvasive, it can be repeated as often as necessary and represents an ideal method to monitor VSP after aneurysmal SAH.

From January 1982 until December 1985 we have evaluated 120 patients with spontaneous SAH by daily measurements of the velocities in the basal cerebral arteries and the internal carotid arteries for 3–4 weeks after the hemorrhage. Details of selected series of these patients have been reported previously (Aaslid 1984, 1986, Seiler 1986). The present report is based on these different series of patients who were mainly operated on after day 10 and who received neither antifibrinolytic drugs nor calcium antagonists. The aim was to study the hemodynamic changes, natural time course and clinical significance of vasospasm after aneurysmal SAH.

Correlation of Flow Velocities with Cerebral Angiography

In 38 patients with a recent SAH the velocities in the middle cerebral arteries (MCAs) and the anterior cerebral arteries (ACAs) were compared with the diameter of these blood vessels as measured from angiograms (Aaslid 1984). The following correlations in the two arteries were found:

1. Middle Cerebral Artery

The normal time-mean velocities in the MCA range from 30–80 cm/sec (Aaslid 1982). MCAs classified as spastic on angiography demonstrated velocities between 120–230 cm/sec. If velocities above 200–250 cm/sec were observed, angiography was postponed for ethical reasons, because in these cases there was probably high grade VSP. Velocities up to 350 cm/sec were seen in single cases. A clear correlation between the velocity of flow and the diameter of the MCA was found (Fig. 1), suggesting that TCD may be used to evaluate VSP of this artery. The MCA is an endartery. Normally there is no, or only limited, collateral circulation by the leptomeningeal anastomosis. Spasm of this artery is therefore a critical condition if the resistance of the narrowed segment increases beyond the compensatory capacity of cerebral autoregulation. Recording of the velocities in both proximal MCAs allows monitoring of VSP after rupture of aneurysms in different locations of the basal arteries, because in multisegmental or global VSP, the proximal part of the MCA is almost always involved (Seiler 1986).

2. Proximal Anterior Cerebral Artery

VSP in this arterial segment is more complicated to assess by TCD. The ACA is less favorably located for Doppler evaluation than the MCA, and recording of velocities in a spastic ACA may be technically difficult. A second problem is the variations in the circle of Willis with hypoplastic

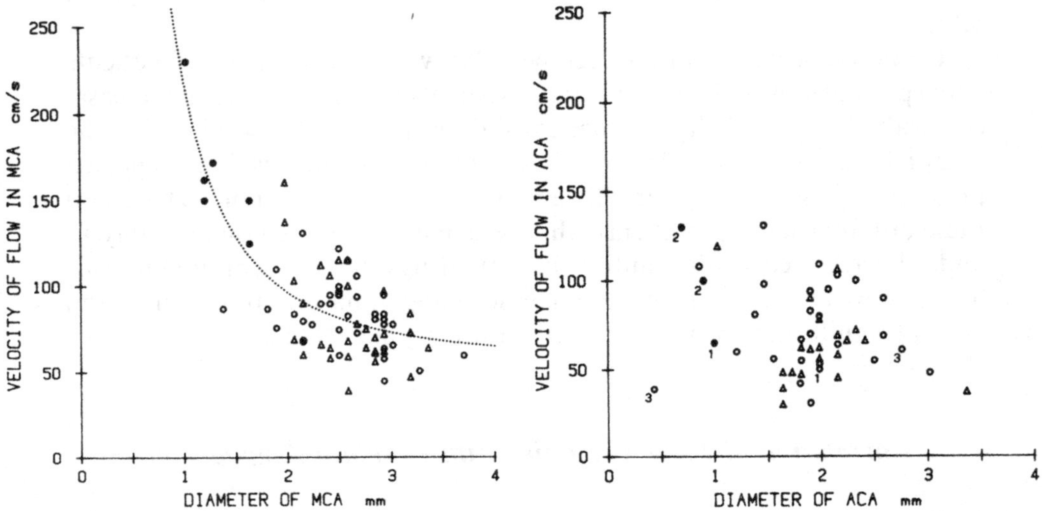

Fig. 1. *Left:* Flow velocity in the middle cerebral arteries (MCAs) as a function of the diameter of that section of the lumen as measured by angiography. Triangles: Cases without angiographic evidence of aneurysm. Circles: Cases with aneurysms. Filled circles: Cases with aneurysms and clear angiographic evidence of vasospasm. The dotted line, $y = 55 + 167/x^2$, was found by nonlinear regression analysis of the entire series. The correlation was $r = 0.75$. *Right:* Flow velocity in the anterior cerebral artery (ACA) as a function of the diameter of that section of the lumen as measured by angiography. Symbols as in left

ACAs. In addition, the proximal ACA is not an end-channel and velocity may be increased because of collateral circulation. Therefore, there is a much higher variability of the flow in the proximal ACAs than in the MCAs. This explains the lack of correlation between diameter and flow velocity in the total series (Fig. 1), which includes a mixture of normal ACAs and bilateral spastic ACAs.

3. Distal ACA and Pericallosal Artery

The segments distal to the anterior communicating artery are normally beyond reach of the present TCD equipment. In cases of symptomatic spasm of both pericallosal arteries, the proximal ACA flow velocity may be only moderately elevated, but often shows a high pulsatility because of the increased peripheral resistance. Also the velocities in the MCAs are not representative enough for the severity of the VSP when the main clot is localized in the pericallosal cistern. Postoperatively after a frontal craniotomy it is possible to monitor the velocities in the pericallosal arteries through a burr hole in the midline.

Secondary Hemodynamic Changes Caused by Cerebral Vasospasm

Musical Murmurs in Cerebral Arteries

In the course of routine recording in patients with spontaneous SAH, we noticed tones of a musical quality from the loudspeaker of the instrument. We realized that an instrument designed to detect Doppler shifts would also act as a demodulator for phase- and amplitude-modulated ultrasonic signals, and thus could be used as a focused microphone. With this approach we observed musical murmurs of pure tone quality in 15 of 32 patients with increased velocities in the cerebral arteries after spontaneous SAH (Aaslid 1984). The frequency range of the pure tones was from 140–820 Hz, corresponding to velocities between 73–215 cm/sec. The maximum amplitude of the musical murmurs was located near the bifurcation of the internal carotid artery (ICA) into MCA and the ACA in the majority of cases. The murmurs occurred as a transitional state between silent, probably laminar flow and the well-known phenomenon of bruit. They were observed between the 4th and the 20th day after SAH. The most likely cause of the musical murmurs is a perodic shedding of vortices, referred to as "a von Karman vortex street". The vortices imply an added mechanical vibrational stress on the arterial wall, and it is uncertain whether the vibrations observed are of sufficient magnitude to have a mechanical influence on the vascular tissue. The clinical significance of the pure tones is related to the development and decay of arterial spasms. The frequency of tones correlates with the degree of spasm, with high frequencies signifying pathologically increased velocities and a narrow arterial lumen.

Reduced Flow Velocity of the Extracranial Internal Carotid Artery

In principle, the flow velocity increase in the cerebral arteries could also be caused by an augmentation in volume flow. In this case the massive increase in the intracranial flow velocities during the second week after SAH should be paralleled by a corresponding trend in the velocities of the extracranial ICA. As expected, however, the latter was significantly reduced in some patients during the period of most severe spasm as a consequence of the increased resistance in the basal cerebral arteries (Aaslid 1986). The extracranial ICA flow velocity was reduced on days 9–15 in the group of patients with intracranial velocities exeeding 200 cm/sec (Fig. 2). This ICA velocity was significantly lower than in the same group during the 4th week when the intracranial velocities had declined.

In the patients with intracranial velocities never exceeding 200 cm/sec, the reduction in ICA velocities during days 9–15 was not statistically significant.

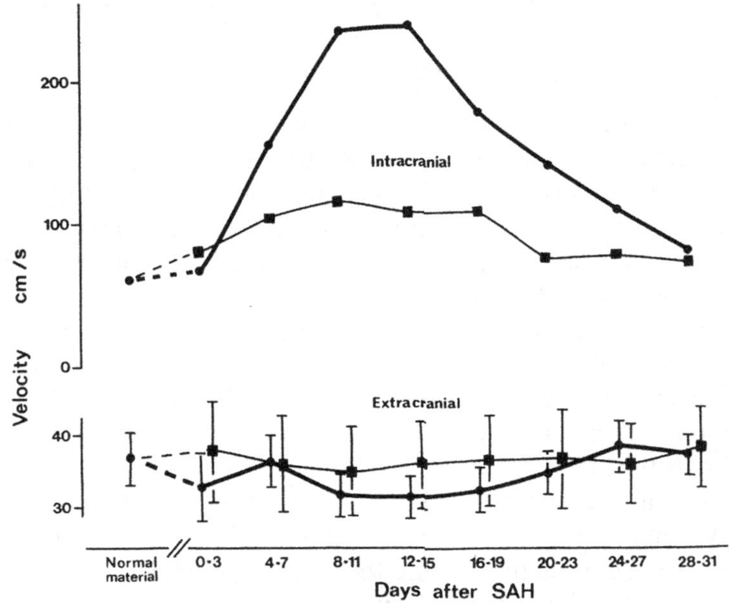

Fig. 2. Comparison of time courses of intracranial and extracranial flow velocities in patients with severe spasm (200 cm/sec, filled circles) and those with only moderate or no spasm (filled squares). The curves represent means of each patient group with bars indicating standard deviations in the lower panel

This can be interpreted as a reduction of CBF by severe VSP and is in accordance with the findings of Meyer *et al.* (1983) using the Xenon inhalation method.

Clinical Significance of Vasospasm Evaluated by TCD

It is important to know the correlation between the change in flow velocity and the course of clinical symptoms. Increase in velocity preceeds clinical symptoms and can therefore be used as a prognostic factor for the management of patients with a spontaneous SAH. For the evaluation of this problem, 39 consecutive patients who were admitted within 10 days after the last SAH were examined daily by TCD for 3–4 weeks. The velocities in both

MCAs were correlated with the clinical status after Hunt and Hess (1968) on the same day (Seiler 1986). Corresponding to the clinical course, the patients were divided in three groups. Group CL 1 (20 patients) had no neurological symptoms, group CL 2 (11 patients) had delayed, but fully reversible neurological symptoms and the patients of group CL 3 (8 cases) suffered a cerebral infarction caused by preoperative VSP. For final analysis a mean

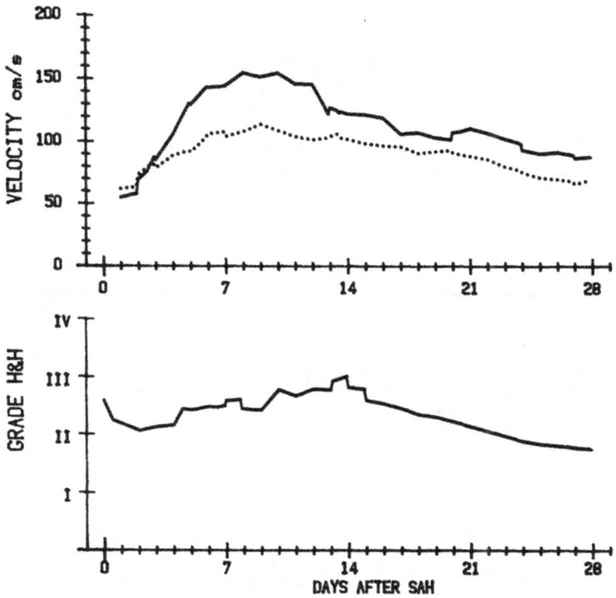

Fig. 3. Mean velocity curve of the side with the higher velocity (continuous line) and the side with the lower velocity (dotted line) correlated with the mean clinical status after Hunt and Hess in 11 patients with transient neurological symptoms. The initial curve shows the natural time course of mild symptomatic vasospasm, because no patient was operated before day 11

velocity curve for both sides and a mean clinical status curve was calculated by computer analysis for each group. The following hemodynamic changes were found in these patients:

Onset and Incidence of Pathological Flow Velocities After SAH

In comparison with 50 healthy adults who had velocities of 62 ± 12 cm/sec in the MCA (Aaslid 1982), we found pathological velocities between 80 and 120 cm/sec in 58% of the patients on the second and third day after the SAH. This early onset of arterial narrowing was not seen angiographically, because MCAs classified as spastic on angiography demonstrated velocities of 120 cm/sec or more (Aaslid 1984). Only two cases had velocities over 120 cm/sec on the third day. It is possible that these patients may have been sensitized by a previous minor bleeding which was not recognized by the referring physician. Clinically important is the fact that patients who later developed brain infarction were characterized by an early and steep increase of the velocity plot. In our opinion, patients with rapidly increasing spasms are particularly vulnerable to an ill-timed operation.

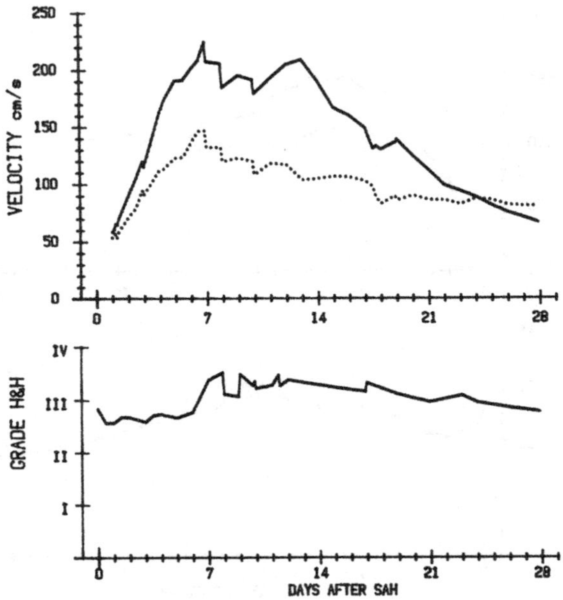

Fig. 4. Mean velocity curve of the side with the higher velocity (continuous line) and the side with the lower velocity (dotted line) correlated with the mean clinical status after Hunt and Hess in 8 patients with permanent neurological symptoms or death due to cerebral infarction. The curve shows the time course of severe symptomatic vasospasm. Note early increase in velocity preceding clinical deterioration

Between days 4 and 10 after SAH we found velocities over 80 cm/sec in the MCAs of all patients of the series. This indicates a higher incidence of VSP evaluated by TCD than seen in angiographic studies (Graf 1974, Sano 1978). Therefore TCD findings of increase velocities can be taken as a diagnostic indicator of SAH in cases of a questionable bleeding.

In laterally localized aneurysms (ICA and MCA) of these series, we found higher velocities on the side of the ruptured aneurysm compared with the nonaffected side in 16 of 18 patients. The difference of the mean velocities was statistically not significant, but this tendency suggests that in bilateral aneurysms where the bleeding side is uncertain from clinical or CT findings, the side of the higher velocity may be taken as an indicator of the ruptured lesion.

Time Course and Correlation with Clinical Status

In the two groups of patients with symptomatic VSP (group CL 2 and CL 3), all operated on after day 10, the mean velocity curves reached their maximum between day 7–12 (Figs. 3 and 4), which corresponds well to the time course of VSP evaluated by angiography (Bergvall 1969, Sano 1978, Weir 1978). There was a direct relation between the severity of the spasm and the steepness of the increase in the velocity (Figs. 3 and 4). The comparison between the velocity and the clinical status curves shows that in

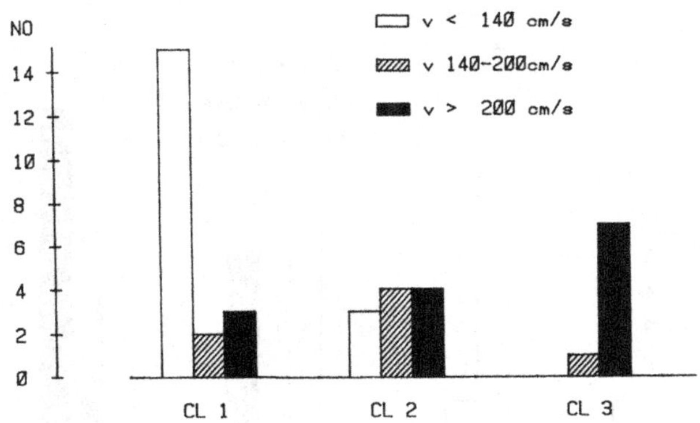

Fig. 5. Distribution of patients with maximal velocity as indicated in the figure within the three clinical groups. Maximal velocity over 200 cm/sec shows a tendency for ischemia, but may remain asymptomatic

symptomatic vasospasm the increase in velocity occurs, as expected, before the manifestation of clinical symptoms. Therefore, Doppler findings can be used as prognostic factors. For clinical purposes we have classified velocities between 140 and 200 cm/sec as moderate spasm and velocities over 200 cm/sec as severe spasm. If we compare the maximum velocity reached in each patient with the clinical status (Fig. 5), it is evident that velocities in the range of 120–140 cm/sec indicate a noncritical state and have never led to brain infarction. Velocities over 200 cm/sec seem to indicate a critical condition with a tendency to ischemia and brain infarction, but they may also remain asymptomatic, probably depending on the existence of collateral circulation and the state of autoregulation of the afflicted region. Especially in such cases, transcranial Doppler ultrasound is of value to detect and monitor this severe but asymptomatic VSP.

Correlation of the Velocity with the CT-visualized Cisternal Blood

A significant correlation between the amount and distribution of subarachnoid blood detected by CT early after aneurysmal rupture and the later development of cerebral VSP visualized angiographically was found by Fisher *et al.* (1980). When there was no subarachnoid blood or it was diffusely distributed, severe VSP was almost never encountered, whereas in the presence of blood clots and thick layers of blood, severe VSP followed almost invariably. These observations have been confirmed by several other authors (Gurusinghe 1984, Mitsukami 1980). In 35 patients who had a CT scan within 5 days after the SAH, we correlated the change in velocities of both MCAs with the CT-visualized subarachnoid blood to investigate if VSP evaluated by TCD has the same positive correlation to the amount of

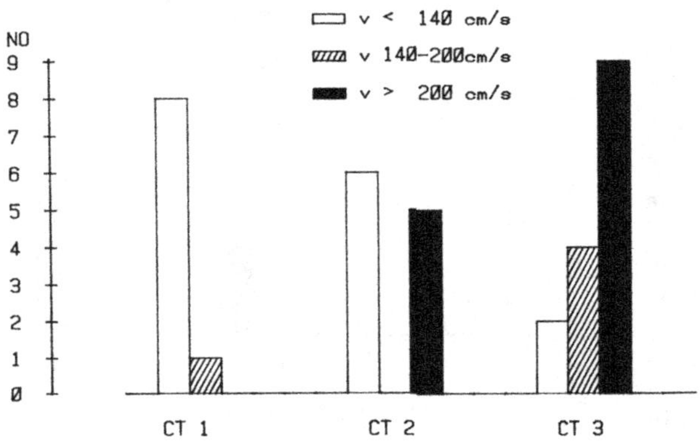

Fig. 6. Distribution of patients with maximal velocity as indicated in the figure within the three CT groups. There is a remarkably positive correlation between the amount of subarachnoid blood and the increase of velocity

cisternal blood as found angiographically (Seiler 1986). The CTs after admission were classified according to the criteria of Fisher *et al.* in three groups. Group CT 1 (9 patients) had a normal CT, group CT 2 (11 patients) showed only diffuse deposits or thin layers of blood and group CT 3 (15 patients) had localized cisternal clots or diffuse thick layers of blood. The maximal velocities recorded in these patients are represented in Fig. 6. There was a significant correlation between the amount of subarachnoid blood and the development of VSP evaluated by TCD. In cases of no, or only little, blood in the basal cisterns (group CT 1 and CT 2) velocities in both MCAs increased only moderately, whereas with the thick clots of subarachnoid blood increase of the velocity with thick clots of subarachnoid blood is in agreement with the observations of Fisher (1980) and others (Gurushinghe 1984, Mitsumaki 1980) that the amount of subarachnoid blood is probably the most important etiological factor for the later development of cerebral vasospasm.

TCD Monitoring in the Management of Patients with Aneurysmal SAH

Timing of Operation

Theoretically, patients with ruptured cerebral aneurysms should be operated on as early as possible to prevent rebleeding, but this is only possible for patients in good condition who are admitted during the first three days after the SAH (Sano 1978, Ljunggren 1981). If they are hospitalized later or in bad condition, most surgeons delay the operation until 10–14 days after the hemorrhage because the operative manipulation may increase VSP, especially during the 4th–7th day after SAH, and lead to postoperative morbidity and mortality (Sano 1978). During this delay the patient may suffer a fatal rebleeding. There is a need for a method that can be used to evaluate for each patient the earliest possible time when the operation can be done without the risk of increasing VSP. The clinical grading as described by Hunt and Hess (1968) is not safe enough because there are patients in grade 1 or 2 who may have severe but asymptomatic VSP (Seiler 1986). A representative case is shown in Fig. 7. With a CT carried out within 5 days after the bleeding (Scotti 1977) patients at high risk for symptomatic VSP due to large cisternal clots or thick layers of subarachnoid blood can be identified (Fisher 1980). But in patients admitted after day 5 or with multiple bleedings, the cisternal blood may be homogenous and with the CT-visualized blood we may evaluate only the risk, but not the actual time course of VSP. Therefore, TCD is an ideal complement to an early CT, because it can be used to monitor onset and resolution of VSP in the individual patient. The noninvasive ultrasonic technique can replace repeated angiographic investigation for this purpose.

In our experience, patients operated during the increasing phase of VSP generally showed a greater increase of the velocities postoperatively. This effect was most significant between days 4–7. In contrast, late surgery during the decreasing phase of the arterial narrowing did not influence the course of VSP very much (Aaslid 1986, Seiler 1986). In the first 3 days after the hemorrhage almost all patients have normal or only slightly increased velocities, therefore TCD plays a minor role in the decision for early operation. In patients admitted later, the time course of VSP should be monitored by TCD during 24–48 hours. If the patients are in grade 1 or 2 and the velocities remain in the range of below 120–140 cm/sec, they should be operated on as early as possible on any day after the hemorrhage. Between days 4–7, the postoperative increase in these patients was never critical and was clinically asymptomatic (Seiler 1986); but in cases with a steep increase of the velocities to subcritical or even critical levels (Fig. 7), angiography and operation should be delayed until decreasing velocities indicate the resolution of VSP.

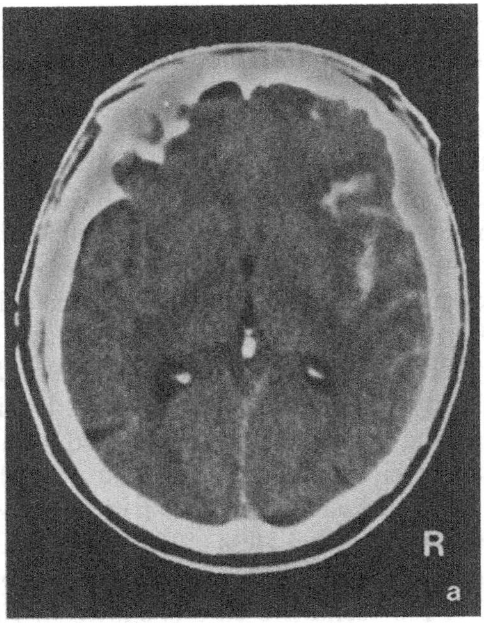

Fig. 7. Illustrative case: Forty-seven year-old man admitted in grade IV after second SAH by rupture of aneurysm of the right middle cerebral artery (MCA). The patient had a first SAH two weeks before. The CT scan after admission is shown in *a*. The MCA Doppler spectra on day 8 are shown in *b*. Severe spasm was suggested by the finding of high velocities (>200 cm/sec) on the right side; this diagnosis was confirmed by the angiogram in *c*. The panel *d* shows how velocities in the right MCA (continuous line) and the left MCA (dotted line) correlated with the clinical status after Hunt and Hess. Note increase of the velocities in right MCA despite clinical improvement of the patient. Operation on day 14 during the decreasing phase of spasm had no significant influence on the velocities. *A* time of angiography, *O* time of surgery

Evaluation of the Effect of Medical Treatment

A large number of agents have been used to prevent or reverse the arterial narrowing, but no means have been definitely identified for treating VSP. Based on the assumption that the final step in all processes leading to arterial smooth muscle contraction is the calcium dependent activation of the actin-myosin complex, the calcium channel blocking agents have received the most contemporary interest, especially the lipid-soluble 1,4-dihydropyridine derivate nimodipine. If this drug has a vasodilating effect on the basal cerebral arteries, the increase of the velocities after SAH should be prevented or reduced.

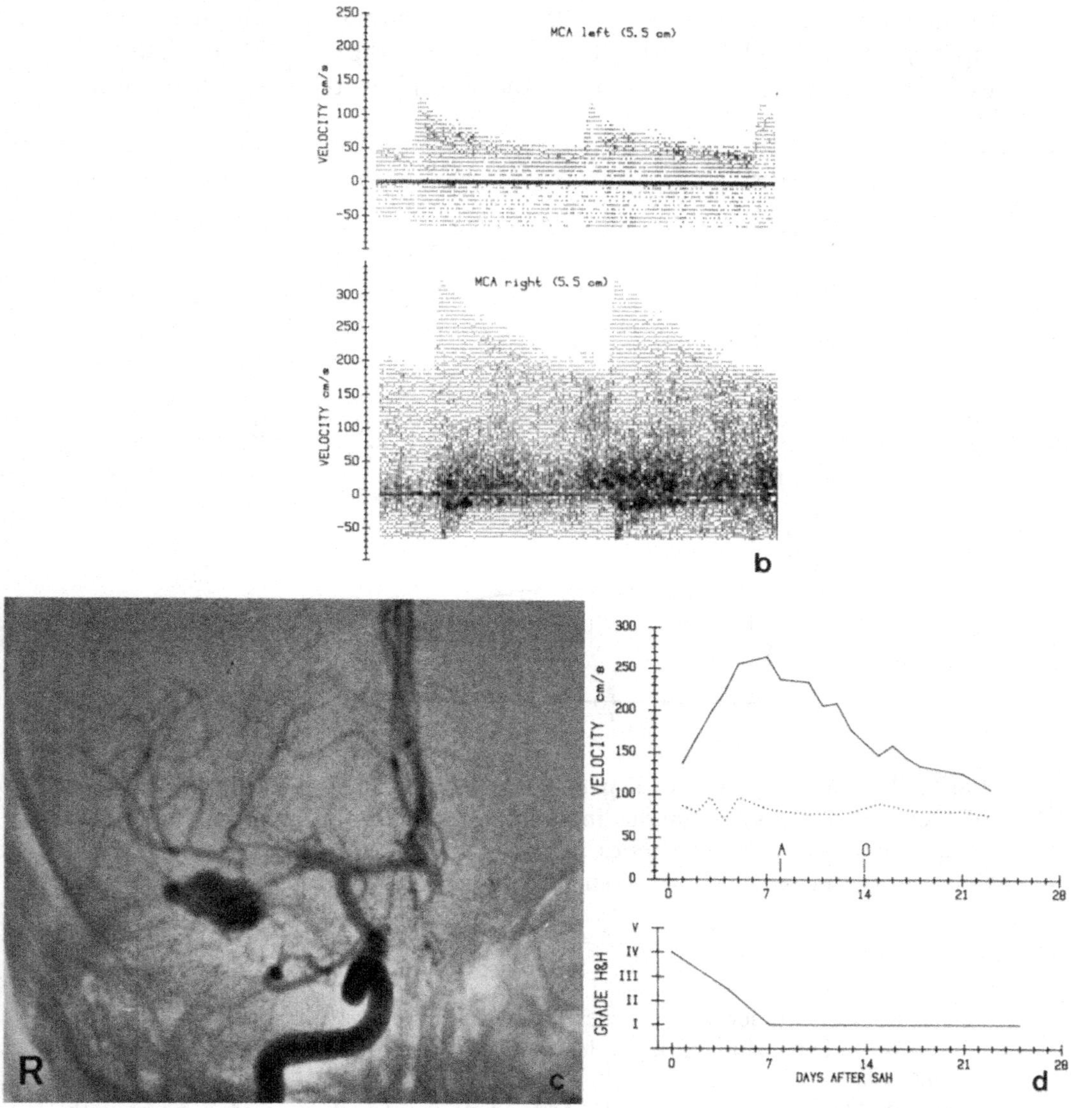

Fig. 7 b–d

In a prospective TCD study, we investigated whether nimodipine administration, started within 4 days after the first SAH, can prevent or diminish the development of chronic VSP evaluated by daily measurements of the BFVs in both MCAs (Seiler 1986). The mean velocity curves of 37 patients treated with nimodipine and of 33 control patients correlated with the mean clinical status after Hunt and Hess are shown in Fig. 8. The velocities are significantly less increased in the nimodipine group compared to the control patients (p = 0.00005). These findings indicate that nimodipine given within 4 days after the SAH does not prevent VSP as evaluated by TCD, but it significantly reduces the severity of the vasoconstriction.

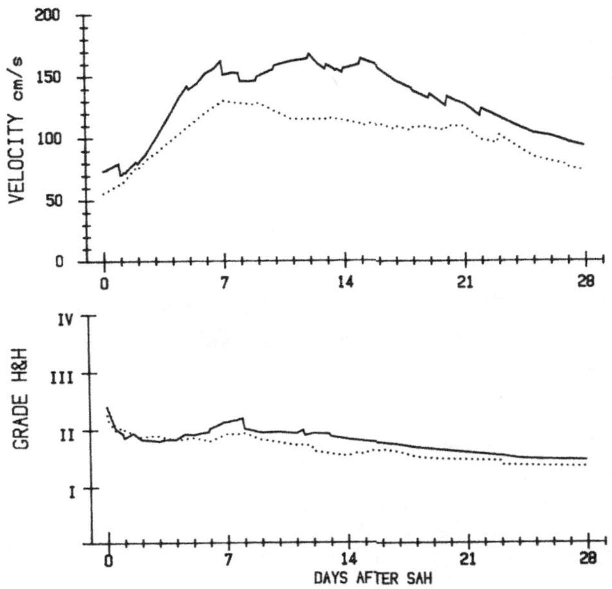

Fig. 8. Mean velocity curves of 37 patients treated with nimodipine (dotted line) and of 33 control patients (continuous line) correlated with the mean clinical status after Hunt and Hess of the two series. There is a statistically significant difference between the nimodipine group and the control patients

References

Aaslid R, Markwalder TM, Nornes H (1982) Noninvasive transcranial Doppler ultrasound recording of flow velocity in basal cerebral arteries. J Neurosurg 57: 769–774

Aaslid R, Huber P, Nornes H (1984) Evaluation of cerbrovascular spasm with transcranial Doppler ultrasound. J Neurosurg 60: 37–41

Aaslid R, Nornes H (1984) Musical murmurs in human cerebral arteries after subarachnoid hemorrhage. J Neurosurg 60: 32–36

Aaslid R, Huber P, Nornes H (1986) A transcranial Doppler method in the evaluation of cerbrovascular spasm. Neuroradiology 28: 11–16

Bergvall U, Galera R (1969) Time relationship between subarachnoid haemorrhage, arterial spasm, changes in cerebral circulation and posthaemorrhagic hydrocephalus. Acta Radiol (Diagn) 9: 229–237

Blaumanis OR, Grady PA, Nelson E (1979) Hemodynamic and morphologic aspects of cerebral vasospasm, In: Price TR, Nelson E (eds) Cerebrovascular diseases. Raven Press, New York, pp 283–294

Ecker A, Riemenschneider PA (1951) Arteriographic demonstration of spasm of the intracranial arteries. With special reference to saccular arterial aneurisms. J Neurosurg 8: 660–667

Fischer CM, Kistler JP, Davis JM (1980) Relation of cerebral vasospasm to subarachnoid hemorrhage visualized by computerized tomographic scanning. Neurosurgery 6: 1–9

Graf CJ, Nibbelink DW (1974) Cooperative study of intracranial aneurysms and subarachnoid hemorrhage. Report on a randomized treatment study. III. Intracranial surgery. Stroke 5: 559–601

Gurusinghe NT, Richardson AE (1984) The value of computerized tomography in aneurysmal subarachnoid hemorrhage. J Neurosurg 60: 763–770

Hughes JT, Schianchi PM (1978) Cerebral artery spasm. A histological study at necropsy of the blood vessels in cases of subarachnoid hemorrhage. J Neurosurg 48: 515–525

Hunt WE, Hess RM (1968) Surgical risk as related to time of intervention in the repair of intracranial aneurysms. J Neurosurg 28: 14–20

Kassell NF, Sasaki T, Colohan ART, Nazar G (1985) Cerebral vasospasm following aneurysmal subarachnoid hemorrhage. Stroke 16: 562–572

Ljunggren B, Brandt L, Kagström E, Sundbärg G (1981) Results of early operations for ruptured aneurysms. J Neurosurg 54: 473–479

Meyer CHA, Lowe D, Meyer M, Richardson PL, Neil-Dwyer G (1983) Progressive change in cerebral blood flow during the first three weeks after subarachnoid hemorrhage. Neurosurgery 12: 58–76

Mitsukami M, Takemae T, Tazawa T, Kawase T, Matsuzaki T (1980) Value of computed tomography in the prediction of cerebral vasospasm after aneurysm rupture. Neurosurgery 7: 583–586

Sano K, Saito I (1978) Timing and indication of surgery for ruptured intracranial aneurysms with regard to cerebral vasospasm. Acta Neurochirurgica 41: 49–60

Scotti G, Ethier R, Melancon D, Terbrugge K, Tschang S (1977) Computed tomography in the evaluation of intracranial aneurysms and subarachnoid hemorrhage. Radiology 123: 85–90

Seiler RW, Grolimund P, Aaslid R, Huber P, Nornes H (1986) Relation of cerebral vasospasm evaluated by transcranial Doppler ultrasound to clinical grade and CT-visualized subrachnoid hemorrhage. J Neurosurg 64 (in press)

Seiler RW, Grolimund P, Zerbrügg H (1986) Evaluation of the calciumantagonist nimodipine for the prevention of vasospasm after aneurysmal subarachnoid hemorrhage. (Submitted for publication)

Weir B, Grace M, Hansen J, Rothberg Ch (1978) Time course of vasospasm in man. J Neurosurg 48: 173–178

Wellum GR, Peterson JW, Zervas NT (1985) The relevance of in vitro smooth muscle experiments to cerebral vasospasm. Stroke 16: 573–581

Author's address: Dr. R. W. Seiler, Neurochirurgische Klinik, Inselspital, CH-3010 Bern, Switzerland.

9. Monitoring Hemodynamic Changes Related to Vasospasm in the Circle of Willis After Aneurysm Surgery

A. Harders

In the last ten years the microneurosurgical treatment of ruptured cerebral aneurysm has become safer, with an operative mortality of 5–7% (Yaşargil 1984). The aim of early surgery within 72 hours after subarachnoid hemorrhage (SAH) is to prevent rebleeding and to be able to start a postoperative medical treatment for vasospasm with hypertonia and/or hypervolemia. The mortality is mainly due to delayed ischemic deficits (DID) with 27% due to vasospasm (Kassell 1984). Because the real cause of vasospasm is not yet known, all therapeutic measures are symptomolytic: either the perfusion pressure of the brain is increased (hypertonia) or the resistance is decreased by preventing the arterial walls from contracting (calcium channel blocker nimodipine) (Allen 1983).

Previously, the time course of vasospasm could only be established by angiography which shows the incidence of vessel diameter reduction (Kodama 1980). With the transcranial Doppler sonographic examination, it is now possible to measure atraumatically and repeatedly individual reaction to arterial narrowing in the brain.

Examination Procedures

Since 1983, we have performed Doppler investigations on patients suffering from SAH. The transcranial Doppler prototype was developed by Aaslid (1982). At intervals of 12 to 36 hours Doppler shift frequencies were recorded in the middle cerebral artery (MCA), supraclinoid portion of the internal carotid artery (ICA), the carotid siphon, the proximal segment of the anterior cerebral artery (A 1), and the posterior cerebral artery (P 1 segment). In special cases, recordings were made in the basilar artery (BA) or in the pericallosal artery (A 2). The prototype instrument had a pulse repetition frequency (PRF) of 8 kHz so that the aliasing effect in "spasm velocities" occurred in measured Doppler shifts above 4 kHz. With a new instrument (TC 2–64 Transcranial Doppler, Eden Medizinische Elektronik,

Ueberlingen, FRG), and a PRF of 10 kHz combined with anti-aliasing techniques, high systolic frequencies up to 10 kHz can be measured (Fig. 12).

Material

A series of 82 patients suffering from SAH were divided into 3 groups:

1. 50 patients undergoing early aneurysm surgery and nimodipine prophylaxis were studied. The locations of the aneurysms are shown in Table 1.

Aneurysm Location	No. of Pats.	Percent
ACoA	23	46
PCoA	4	8
MCA	13	26
ACA (A 2)	2	4
AChorA	2	4
ICA Bif	3	6
Multiple	2	4
PICA	1	2
Total	50	100

Table 2. *Preoperative clinical grading according to Hunt and Hess scale*

Grade		n	%
I	asymptomatic or minimal headache and slight nuchal rigidity	3	6
II	moderate to severe headache, nuchal rigidity, no neurological deficit other than cranial nerve palsy	15	30
III	drowsiness, confusion or mild focal deficit	21	42
IV	stupor, moderate to severe hemiparesis, possibly early decerebrate rigidity, and vegetative disturbances	11	22
V	deep coma, decerebrate rigidity, moribund appearance	0	0
	Total	50	100

2. 12 patients with SAH but without surgery.

3. In 20 patients on which surgery was performed later than 72 hours following SAH.

The preoperative neurological grading (Hunt and Hess 1968) correlated with the amount of blood in the subarachnoid space (Table 2).

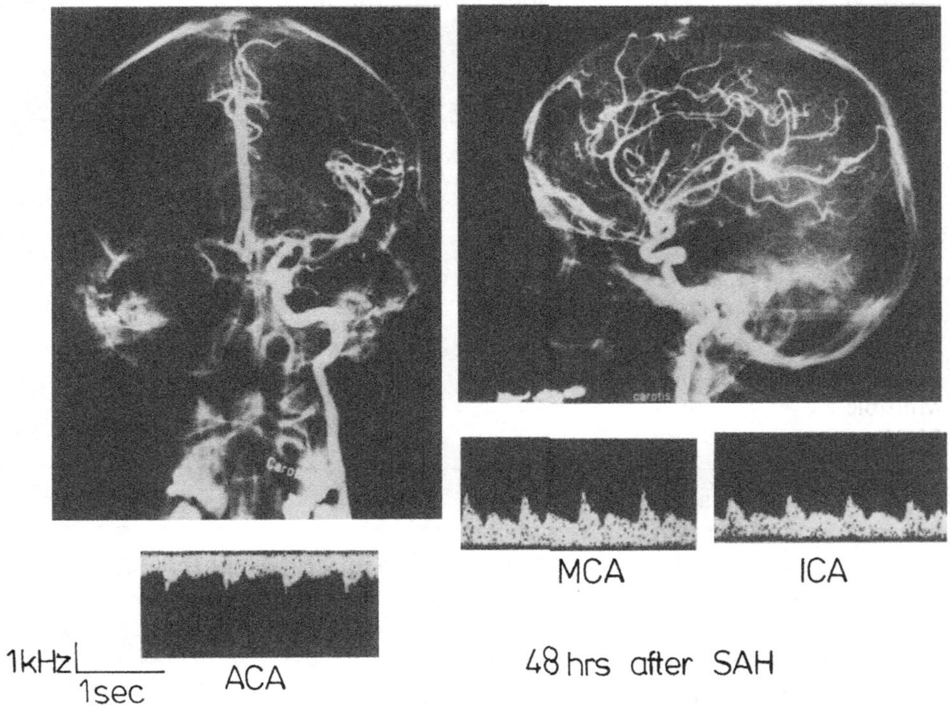

Fig. 1. Forty-eight hours after SAH from a ACoA aneurysm, angiography shows no vasospasm. Transcranial Doppler frequencies and flow patterns are normal

The mean values of the frequencies measured on each day were calculated for each of the groups (expressed in kHz from the time average outline frequencies).

Hemodynamic Changes in the Circle of Willis After SAH and Early Aneurysm Operation

Hemodynamic Changes in the First 72 Hours After SAH

In 40 patients, Doppler frequencies could be correlated with vessel diameter determined by angiography within the first 3 days after SAH. In no case were there increased velocities, and angiography showed no spasm. The

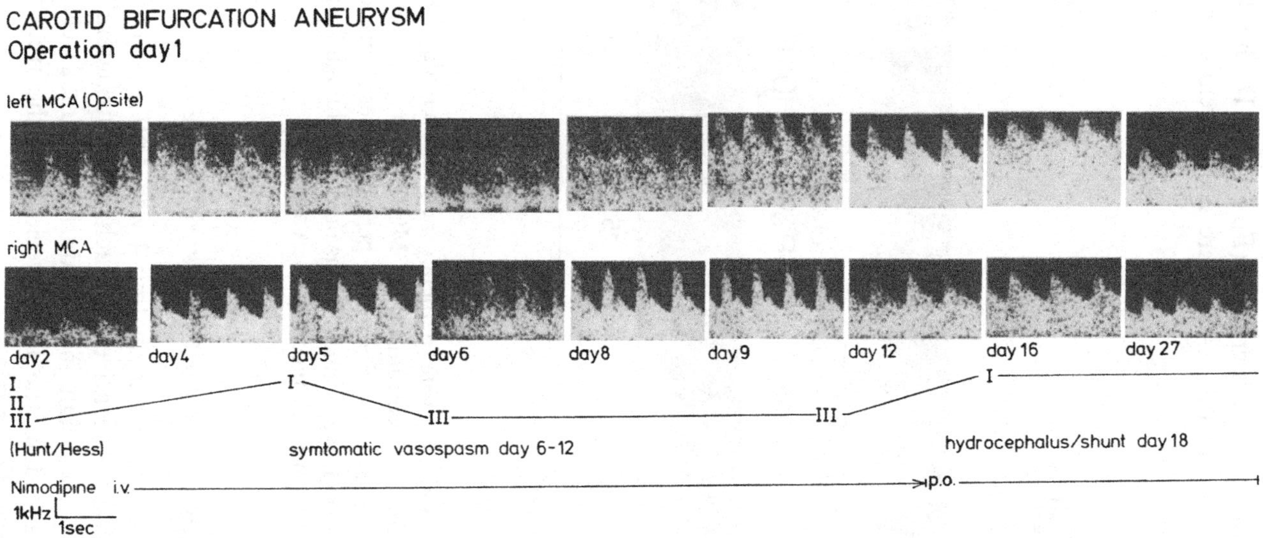

Fig. 2. Time course of frequency changes in both MCAs after early operation and nimodipine treatment. Severe frequency increase in the left MCA resulting from symptomatic vasospasm with delayed ischemic deficit from day 6 to day 12. Moderate (subcritical) vasospasm of the contralateral MCA. In both arteries slight acceleration (day 16) after changing from intravenous to oral nimodipine administration

arteries appeared dilated (Fig. 1). The frequency range in the MCA was 1.3–1.7 kHz, in the ICA 1.4–1.7 kHz.

These findings confirm the intraoperative Doppler values described by Gilsbach (1983), and reports in the literature (Fox 1978, Hashii 1972) indicate that in the first 3 days after SAH there is hyperemia and no vasospasm.

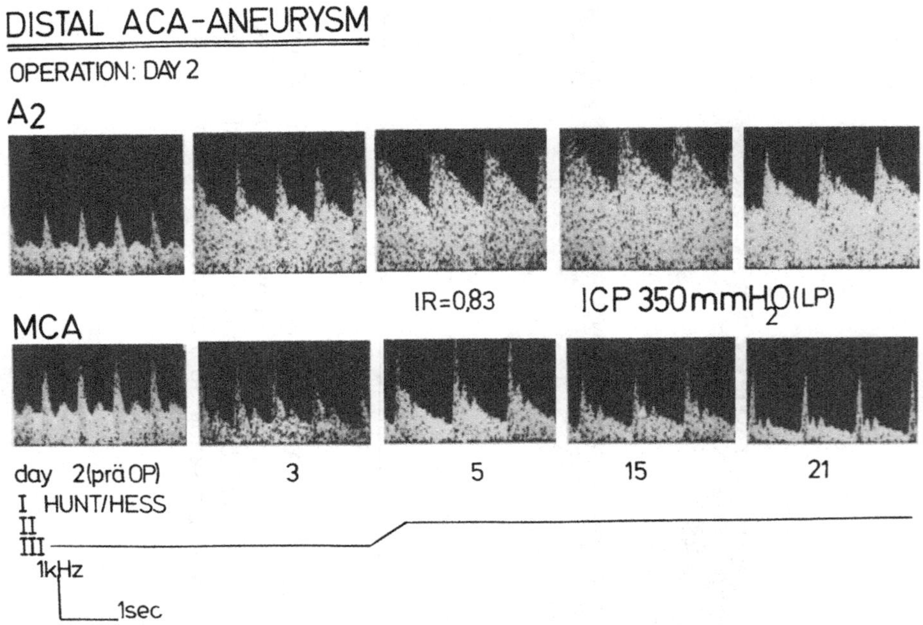

Fig. 3. Subcritical vasospasm and moderate frequency increase up to day 15 in the pericallosal artery. The frequency spectrum of the MCA (during operation no splitting of the Sylvian fissure) indicates increased peripheral resistance due to spinal fluid flow disturbance. Improved clinical status on day 5, though frequency and index of resistance had increased

Hemodynamic Changes from Day 4 to the Following 6 Months

Typical changes in individual frequency within 4 weeks after SAH in the MCA and the A 2 on the side of operative approach and contralaterally are shown in Figs. 2 and 3. There is a slight increase during the first 2 weeks, the maximum level being reached in the third week, with the frequencies returning to normal in the next 4 weeks.

The time of the frequency changes due to vasospasm in the different arteries of 50 patients (group 1) are summarized in Figs. 4 and 5: The greatest hemodynamic effect occurred in the MCA and the ICA, in contrast

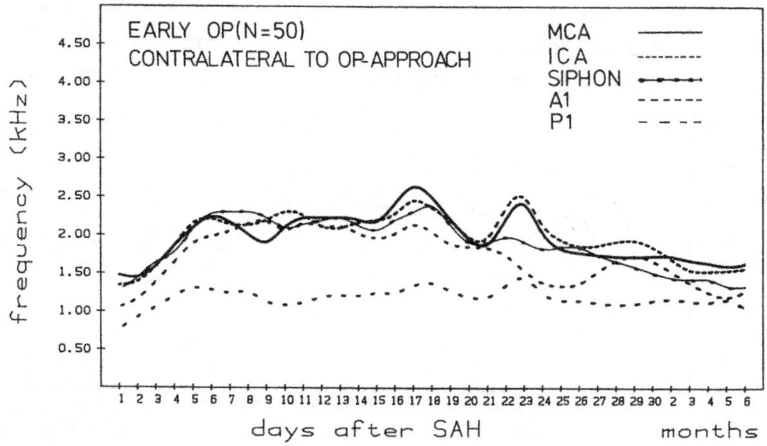

Fig. 4

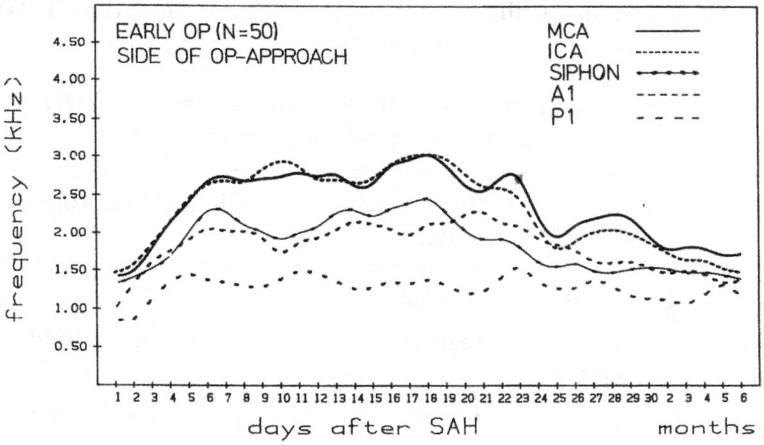

Fig. 5

Figs. 4 and 5. Time course of frequency changes in the MCA, the ICA, the siphon, the A 1 and the P 1 on the side of operative approach and contralaterally in 50 patients. Increase in the first 10 days, then maximum level up to days 18–19, then decrease. On the side where the Sylvian fissure was split, frequencies are higher (Fig. 5)

to less reaction in the A 1 and P 1. Frequencies on the operated side were always higher than on the contralateral side.

Cases with severe SAH developed more spasm than those with slight SAH (Fig. 6).

Delayed Ischemic Deficits

Eight patients developed delayed ischemic deficits (DID) in the second week after SAH. The frequency changes in the MCA showed a rapid increase to

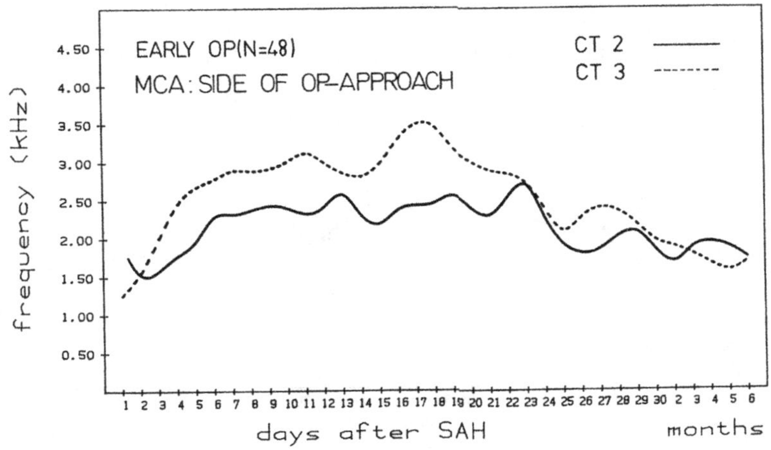

Fig. 6. Patients with severe SAH and thick blood layers in all basal cisterns (CT III) show increased hemodynamic changes compared with moderate SAH (CT II) in the first 3 weeks

Table 3. *Flow pattern, blood flow velocity, and clinical significance for patients suffering SAH* and developing vasospasm*

Type	Flow velocity**	Flow pattern	Clinical Importance
Normal	< 2 kHz	regular	
Unspecific Acceleration	~ 2 kHz	regular	must be controlled
Subcritical Spasm	2–3 kHz	regular	preventive therapy
Critical Spasm	> 3 kHz	irregularities, wall artefacts	symptomatic therapy

* For ICA, MCA, ACA; ** Time averaged peak frequency.

more than 3 kHz within the first 6 days, while patients without neurological deficits never reached more than 3 kHz (averaged values). Based on these findings the frequencies were related to the degree of spasm in clinical practice as shown in Table 3 and Fig. 7.

Hemodynamic Changes Due to Nimodipine

In 33 patients the calcium channel blocker nimodipine was given intravenously (2 mg/h) for 14 days and orally for a further 6 days (4 × 60 mg). The

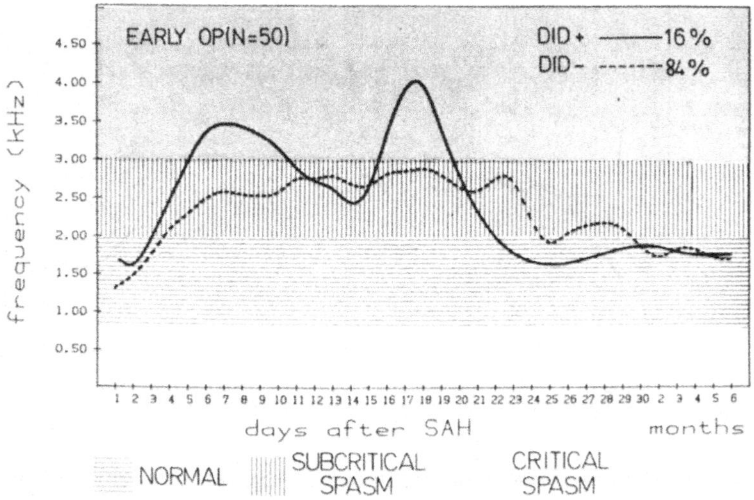

Fig. 7. Rapid frequency increase in the first 6 days to more than 3 kHz indicates an ischemic risk for the patient. The double peak frequency course may be caused by changes in nimodipine administration. Clinically the delayed ischemic deficit (DID) group had reversible neurological deficits in the second week after SAH

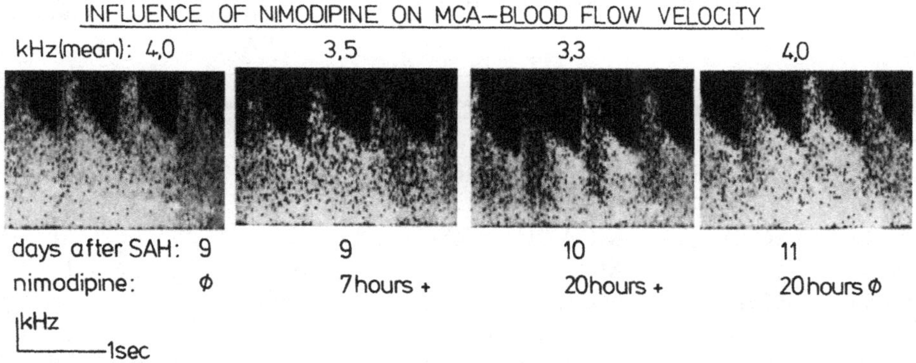

Fig. 8. Frequency changes after nimodipine administration. A marked decrease is observed 7 and 20 hours after starting infusion. Stopping the infusion reverses this trend, as shown in the right panel

frequencies in the MCA dropped shortly before days 14 and 21, with a secondary increase following each reduction. These frequency changes when the mode of drug application is changed can only be explained by the vasodilatory effect (Figs. 8 and 9). Five patients had received no nimodipine prophylaxis and the frequencies in the MCA in these patients showed higher levels compared to the nimodipine group.

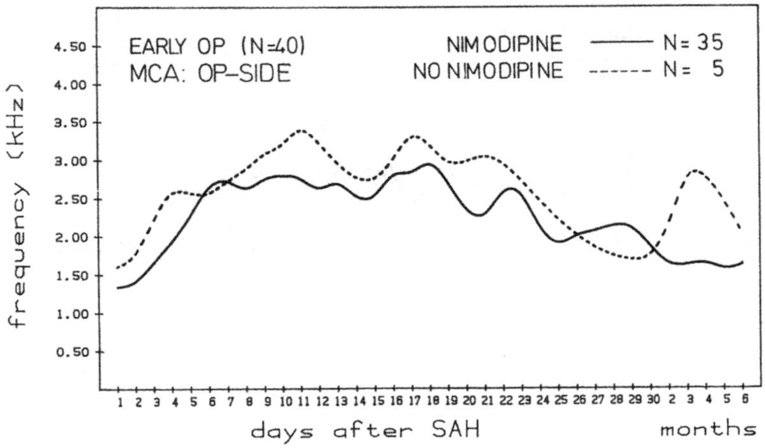

Fig. 9. Patients without nimodipine treatment (n = 5) show higher frequencies than treated patients

Table 4. *Location, occurrence, and duration of musical murmurs as a sign of severe vasospasm*

Pat.	Aneurysm	Location of MM	Occurrence of MM (Days after SAH)	Re-cording Days
f 37	ICA (L)	MCA/ICA (L)	8	5
m 25	MCA (L)	MCA (L)	8	16
f 53	MCA (R)	MCA/ICA (R)	5	6
f 47	MCA (R)	MCA (R)	10	3
f 54	ACoA (r)	MCA/ICA (R)	12	1
m 34	ACoA (r)	MCA/ICA (R)	6	18
f 56	ACoA (r)	MCA (R) ACoA (A 1) (L)	~ 5 weeks	
m 70	MCA (R)	MCA (R)	4	19
f 59	MCA (L)	MCA (L)	6	3
m 28	ACoA (1)	MCA/ICA (L)	6	4
m 45	PCoA (R)	MCA/ICA/A 1 (R)	7	2
f 65	PCoA (R)	MCA (R)	7	2
m 22	ICA (R)	MCA/ICA/A 1 (R)	8	12
f 38	PICA (L)	ICA (R)	11	2
m 51	MCA (R)	ICA (L)	6	1
f 39	ACoA (r)	ICA (R)	10	1
f 34	PCoA (L)	ICA/A 1 (L)	6	2
f 54	ICA (R)	ICA (L)	14	2

R/L = Location of aneurysm; r/l = Side of operative approach

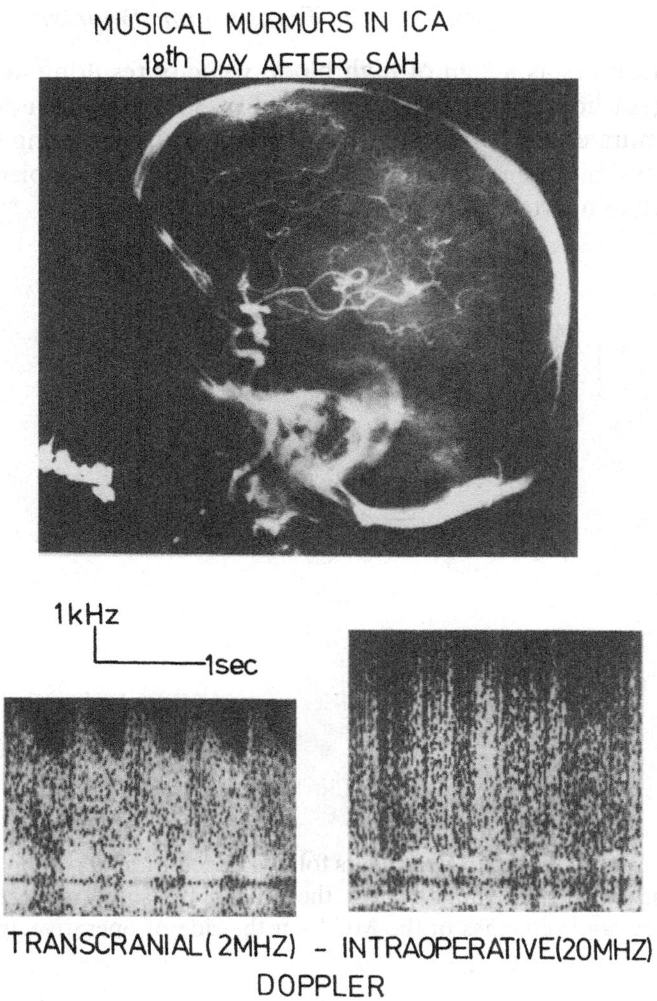

Fig. 10. Angiographically, the distal segment of the ICA has a slight spasm of about 50% diameter reduction. In transcranial Doppler 3.5-fold increase of diastolic velocity and musical murmurs. Intraoperative Doppler confirms musical murmurs caused by an arteriosclerotic plaque and spasm

Intracerebral Hemorrhage and Vasospasm

What is the effect of intracerebral hemorrhage following aneurysm rupture? A comparison of the frequency changes in the MCA on the operated side in 6 patients undergoing surgery for MCA aneurysm and intracerebral hematoma, and those of 11 patients with severe SAH from a midline aneurysm (ACoA) showed that the time maximum frequency was reached one week later in the hematoma group.

Musical Murmurs in Transcranial Doppler

Musical murmurs as a sign of high blood velocity resulting in vessel wall vibration (Aaslid 1984) could be recorded in 36% of the cases (Table 4). Such murmurs could be recorded more often with increasing experience. Fig. 10 shows this phenomenon not only in transcranial Doppler but also in intraoperative microvascular Doppler (20 MHz).

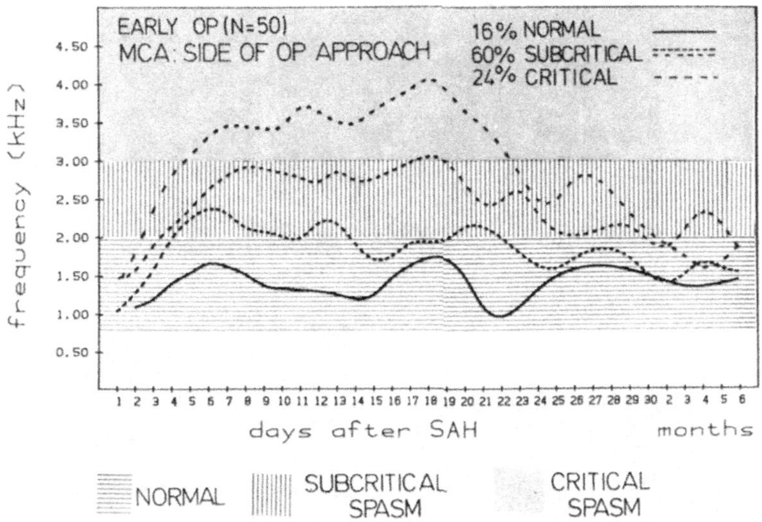

Fig. 11. Frequency ranges in 50 patients following acute aneurysm operation. Only 16% are in the normal range, whilst the other 84% show moderate or severe hemodynamic changes in the MCA on the side of operative approach

Grading of Spasm

What is the incidence of hemodynamic changes in patients suffering SAH who are treated by early operation and nimodipine prophylaxis? In 16% there was only a slight increase up to 2 kHz, which we call nonspecific acceleration (Fig. 11). In 26% the mean Doppler shift increased to between 2 and 3 kHz—clinically categorized as subcritical spasm. In 36% there was an increase up to between 3 and 4 kHz and in 24% up to more than 4 kHz. The upper frequency range was found to be correlated to critical spasm.

Hemodynamic Changes and Surgery

Fig. 13 shows the time course of the frequency changes in the MCA in 12 patients without aneurysm surgery (group 2). The increase occurs up to day

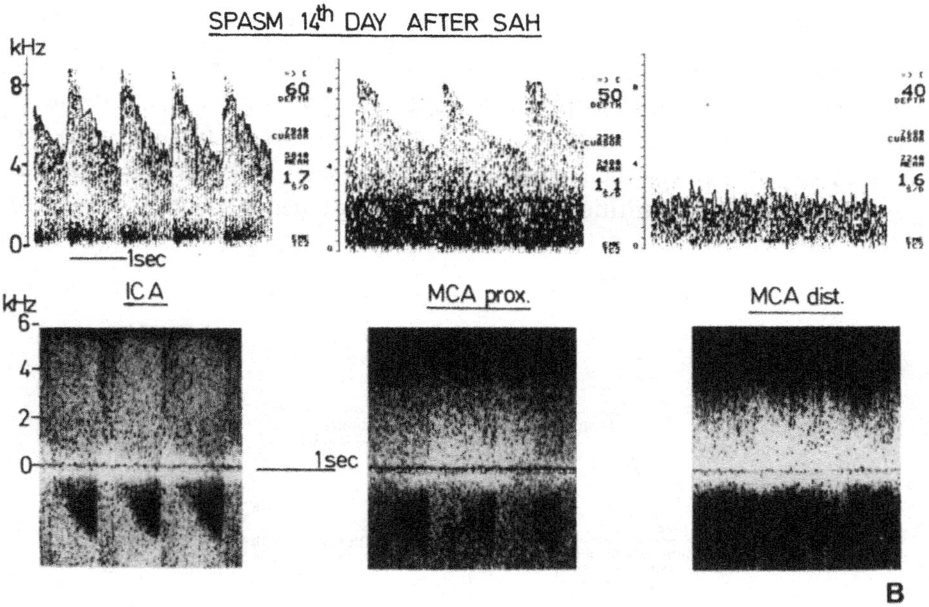

Fig. 12. *A* Frequency spectra recorded with the new TC 2–64 with a pulse repetition frequency up to 10 kHz and antialiasing. *B* Frequency spectra with the prototype transcranial Doppler and a pulse repetition frequency of 8 kHz

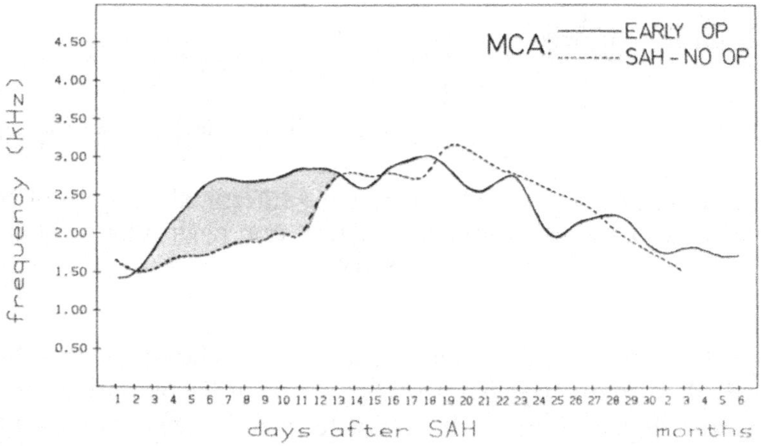

Fig. 13. Only in the first 12 days is there a different rate of frequency increase in the time course of patients with early surgery (n = 50) and patients without surgery (n = 20)

16–20 as in the operated group. The highest values are found in MCA, ICA and siphon (3.5 kHz), with the lowest values in A 1 and P 1.

Twenty patients were operated on later than 72 hours after SAH (group 3). Angiography or surgery was performed only when the highest frequency in the circle of Willis was below 3 kHz (1 case had 3.5 kHz).

Discussion

Transcranial Doppler is the first suitable method for evaluating the hemodynamic effect of vasospasm. Angiography, with increased morbidity risk of up to 5–10 times in spasm, is no longer necessary in such cases. In early aneurysm surgery the individual time course of Doppler shift changes was measured and the influence of the following parameters established: In

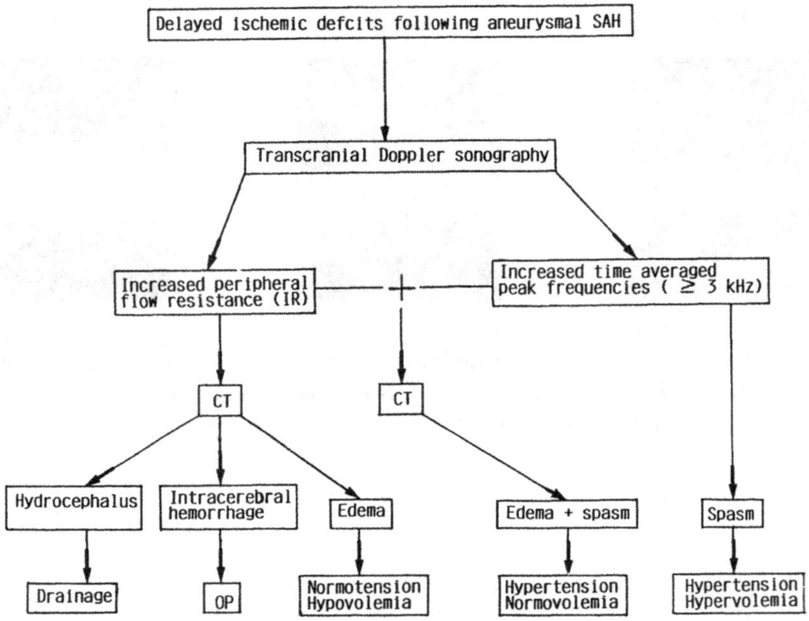

Fig. 14. The value of transcranial Doppler in the differential diagnosis of delayed ischemic deficits following aneurysmal SAH. Repeat angiography is no longer necessary

the first 3 days there is hyperemia but no spasm. The MCA and the ICA show the highest frequency changes. On the side of the operative approach, velocities were higher than on the opposite side. This contradicts the view that removing the blood in the subarachnoid space reduces the severity of the spasm. The maximum of vasospasm in our series was not around the 7th to 10th day as reported by Kassell (1982) but between the 17th and 21st day.

Aneurysm surgery does not appear to influence the maximum value of the frequencies but rather the time it takes for the maximum to be reached (Fig. 13). The severity of the vasospasm depends on the amount of subarachnoid blood. There are two possible effects producing changes in frequencies after changing the form of nimodipine administration: 1. dilatation of the small resistance vessels with increase of collateral flow, and

2. dilatation of the large spastic basal arteries. If all the small resistance vessels increased in diameter, the velocity measured in the MCA or the ICA due to diminished peripheral resistance would increase and not decrease; therefore, the last effect seems to predominate. Increasing perfusion pressure by induced hypertonia results in decrease of Doppler shift (Fig. 15). The investigation procedure in patients developing DID is shown

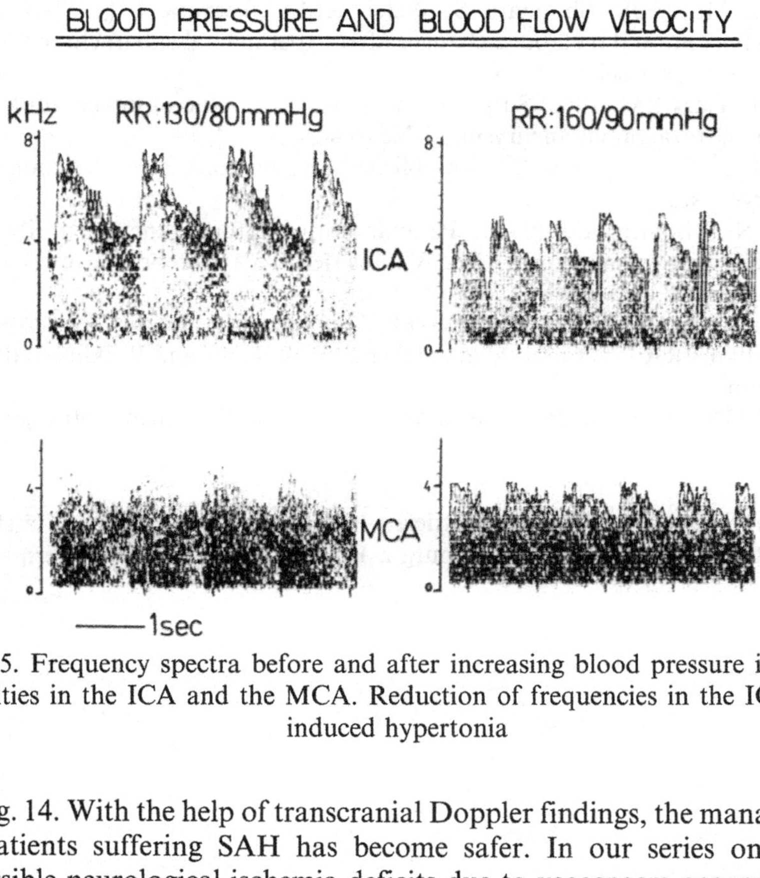

Fig. 15. Frequency spectra before and after increasing blood pressure in spasm velocities in the ICA and the MCA. Reduction of frequencies in the ICA after induced hypertonia

in Fig. 14. With the help of transcranial Doppler findings, the management of patients suffering SAH has become safer. In our series only 14% reversible neurological ischemia deficits due to vasospasm occurred. One patient (2%) died of ischemic brain infarction due to insufficient blood pressure management in vasospasm though established by Doppler investigation.

References

Aaslid R, Markwalder T-M, Nornes H (1982) Noninvasive transcranial Doppler ultrasound recording of flow velocity in basal cerebral arteries. J Neurosurg 57: 769–774

Aaslid R, Huber P, Nornes H (1984) Evaluation of cerebrovascular spasm with transcranial Doppler ultrasound. J Neurosurg 60: 37–41

Aaslid R, Nornes H (1984) Musical murmurs in human cerebral arteries after subarachnoid hemorrhage. J Neurosurg 60: 32–36

Allen GS *et al* (1983) Cerebral arterial spasm—a controlled trial of nimodipine in patients with subarachnoid hemorrhage. New Engl J Med 38: 619–624

Fox JL, Ko JP (1978) Cerebral vasospasm: A clinical observation. Surg Neurol 10: 269–275

Gilsbach JM (1983) Intraoperative Doppler sonography in neurosurgery. Springer, Wien New York

Hashi K, Meyer JS, Shinmaru S, Welch KMA, Teraura T (1972) Cerebral hemodynamic and metabolic changes after experimental subarachnoid hemorrhage. J Neurol Sci 17: 1–14

Hunt WE, Hess RM (1968) Surgical risk as related to time of intervention in the repair of intracranial aneurysms. J Neurosurg 28: 14–19

Kassell NF, Torner JC (1982) Unpublished observations from the cooperative aneurysm study

Kassell NF, Boarini DJ (1980) Patients with ruptured aneurysm: Pre- and postoperative management. In: Wilkins RA (ed) Cerebral arterial spasm. Williams and Wilkins, Baltimore London

Kodama N, Mizoi K, Sakurai Y, Suzuki J (1980) Incidence and onset of vasospasm. In: Wilkins RA (ed) Cerebral arterial spasm. Williams and Wilkins, Baltimore London

Yaşargil GM (1984) Microneurosurgery, vols I and II. Thieme, Stuttgart New York

Author's address: Dr. A. Harders, Neurochirurgische Universitätsklinik, Hugstetter Strasse 55, D-7800 Freiburg i. Br., Federal Republic of Germany.

10. Transcranial Doppler Monitoring

E. B. Ringelstein

Introduction

The monitoring concept in neurology, neurosurgery and vascular surgery refers to the continuous or intermittent evaluation of nervous and/or circulatory functions in order to detect otherwise obscure alterations of the patient's condition. The underlying idea is that monitoring delivers immediate information about potential hazards or the effectiveness of interventions and thus may lead to rapid modifications of therapy. Monitoring of representative parameters is of particular interest if the desired information cannot be acquired with more common methods, for instance, by clinical examination of the patient. This is why monitoring techniques are predominantly applied in non-cooperative or comatose patients. This is particularly the case in the operating room, during intensive care and neuroradiological or surgical interventions, where immediate information about the induced changes in the patient's state is lacking (Hacke 1985, Ringelstein *et al.* 1985 b, Ringelstein *et al.* 1986).

In the past, any alteration of the cerebral circulation could not be detected except by means of repeat angiography or blood flow measurements which had to be performed in an off-line fashion. Such studies have been used, for instance, in patients with increased ICP (Obrist *et al.* 1979), following vasospasm due to subarachnoid hemorrhage (Mickey *et al.* 1984), during open-heart surgery (Henriksen *et al.* 1983), vascular reconstruction of the brain supplying arteries (Sundt *et al.* 1981) and occluding or dilating neuroradiological interventions. This kind of examination should not be regarded as monitoring in a strict sense, as the data had to be stored for later interpretation. In any case, there is a considerable delay in the output of clinically useful information.

Electrophysiological parameters have the disadvantage of being only indirect and also somewhat delayed indicators of brain ischemia and are burdened with the difficulties of their formal interpretation, particulary under general anesthesia (Markand *et al.* 1984). Additionally, electrophysical parameters do not allow for precise grading of the severity of the impairment of cerebral blood supply. Once the critical threshold is breached, evoked potentials or EEG will become severely affected without indicating whether there is still a reversible functional disturbance or already an irreversible ischemic brain damage (Jacobs *et al.* 1983).

Transcranial Doppler sonography (TCD) compensates for some of these shortcomings in that it *immediately* reflects the *true* circulatory conditions within the insonated arteries. One of the most important determinants of outcome in partial ischemic states is residual perfusion. This can be continuously quantified with the help of TCD, allowing timely intervention if necessary. Although TCD only records the mean flow velocity of the blood column, this parameter very closely reflects the true volume flow when compared with electromagnetic or CBF measurements (Ries *et al.* 1985, Lundar *et al.* 1985).

TCD meets the basic criteria of a useful monitoring technique. Apart from being completely noninvasive, the cerebral artery flow velocities are available immediately. Individual baseline recordings can be performed preoperatively to find out whether monitoring of a certain artery is possible or not (see Chapter 3).

This also allows for preoperative assessment of the ideal position of both the probe and the sample volume (Ringelstein *et al.* 1985 b).

Data can be obtained continuously. Monitoring does not interfere with or prolong the operative procedure. TCD-monitoring findings may initiate rapid modifications of therapy, for instance insertion of a shunt, better adaption of extracorporeal blood pumping, deflation of balloon cathethers, etc.

At the moment, TCD monitoring cannot be replaced by simpler methods. TCD monitoring equipment is small and mobile. Apart from deterioration of the flow signal by thermocautery applications, there is no limitation for use of TCD neither in the operating room nor in the intensive care unit.

Up to now, there is only very limited experience with TCD-monitoring in the various clinical settings. This is why the following report is primarily based on the author's personal experience. However, the results of other groups will also be included as far as they have already been published in papers or communicated verbally.

Technical Equipment

Initially, our studies were performed with a prototype of the transcranial Doppler device. Later, a serial TC2-64 device was used [Eden Medizinische Elektronik (EME), D-7770 Ueberlingen, Federal Republic of Germany]. For better photographic documentation of the flow signals, an Angioscan

FFT-spectrum analyzer was also used and a commercial tape deck was added for analog storage of the signals. During playback, the flow signals could be displayed in order to freeze the interesting phases of the procedure on the Angioscan for scientific illustrations. However, this time-consuming technique is no longer necessary. The standard version of the transcranial Doppler device (TC 2-64) allows for a wide-range variation of both the time scales as well as the amplitude of the signal.

Most of our studies have been performed with hand-held positioning of

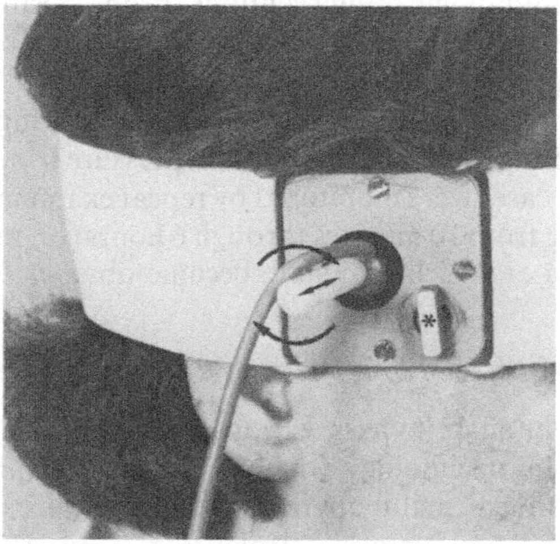

Fig. 1. Prototype flat transcranial Doppler probe (EME Ueberlingen, type FP 2) mounted in the temporal region during insonation of the MCA. The probe can freely be adjusted within its frame as indicated by arrows and can be fixed by turning the switch (asterisk). The adjusting handle is removable

the probe during the whole intervention under study. Meanwhile, a much more comfortable surveillance of intracranial blood flow velocity has become possible with the help of a flat probe, fixed preoperatively in the temporal region of the skull (type FP 2; EME, Ueberlingen, FRG) (Fig. 1). The mechanical construction of the probe allows for an individual adaption of the insonation angle. The point of penetration (window) can be selected by moving the entire assembly on the temporal surface. As soon as the ideal position of the probe is achieved it can be firmly fixed by clamping within the frame.

Insonation Technique

In order to obtain a representative parameter of the global hemispheric blood flow, the proximal stem (M1 segment) of the MCA is insonated via a transtemporal approach. It is wise to find the ideal position of the probe (*i.e.*, site of the ultrasound window within the temporal skull) and the optimal position of the sample volume (*i.e.*, insonation depth with the strongest flow signal) preoperatively. Perioperatively, the same probe position and insonation depth should be used. In most cases, the temporal ultrasound window is situated immediately anterior and superior to the tragus of the ear conch. The optimal insonation depth depends on the transverse diameter of the skull (Ringelstein and Kahlscheuer, unpublished data). Usually, a distinct MCA flow signal can be achieved at 50, 55 or 60 mm.

During neuroradiological interventions, probe positioning depends on the vascular territory under study. So far we have predominantly used the transtemporal approach (Ringelstein *et al.* 1985 c).

With the new probe described, *continuous* monitoring is now facilitated in patients exhibiting increased intracranial pressure from whatever reason. Previously, these cases were monitored by repeat examinations in very short intervals (ranging from 10 minutes through 6 hours) or, at least, as soon as a critical alteration of the clinical state became obvious (see below).

Monitoring of MCA Flow Velocity During Open-Heart Surgery

During cardiopulmonary bypass, extracorporeal oxygenation of the blood requires a pumping technology which severely alters physiological blood flow. During artificial maintainance of the arterial circulation, hypoxic brain damage and perioperative stroke may occur (Furlan and Breuer 1984). Transcranial Doppler monitoring of the MCA flow velocity may indicate whether cerebral blood supply is sufficient or not. However, the ischemic threshold is not yet known, neither individually nor in general. At the moment, the aim of TCD monitoring during open heart surgery is fourfold, namely 1. to analyze the presumed dissociation of the flow-metabolism junction, 2. to identify the hazards of accidental *hyper*perfusion, 3. to maintain sufficient MCA flow velocities which are known to be on the safe side of a critical perfusion pressure and 4. to evaluate empirically the lower limit of still tolerable flow reduction. Presumably, TCD will allow for a more precise adaption of the heart-lung machine to the patient's demands in order to prevent postoperative encephalopathy. Doppler measurements should at least be taken at short intervals. During critical maneuvers, continuous monitoring is preferable. Preoperatively, TCD helps to identify patients at high risk for ischemic encephalopathy with the help of a CO_2-inhalation test by assessing the autoregulatory capacity of the brain arterioles (Ringelstein *et al.* 1985 a, Grosse *et al.* 1985). Apart from a few personal experiences with intraoperative MCA flow monitoring during open heart surgery (Fig. 2), von Reutern and his group (1985) have recently elaborated some basic data obtained during 17 operations. The mean MCA

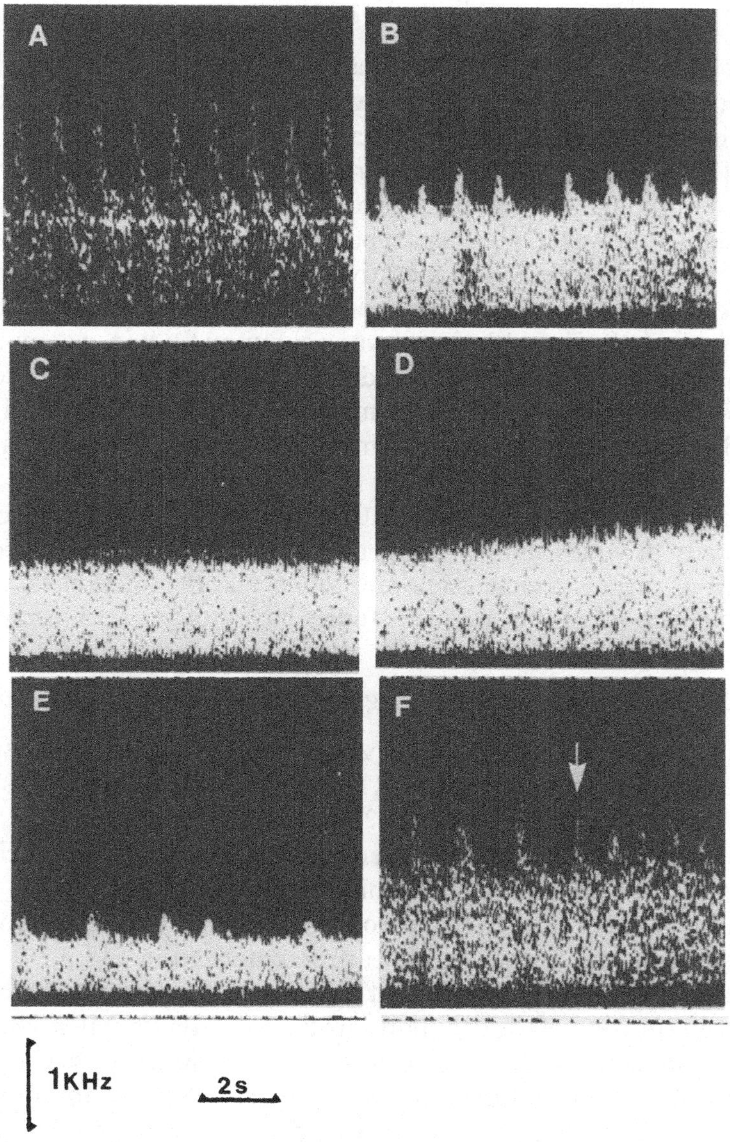

Fig. 2. Different phases of MCA flow velocity monitoring during cardiopulmonary bypass. *A* Normal MCA flow signals immediately after establishment of general anesthesia. *B* High continuous diastolic flow velocity after starting the heart-lung machine. Systolic velocity peaks due to residual spontaneous myocardial contractions are still visible. *C* Nonpulsatile MCA flow velocity during extracorporeal oxygenation. *D* The pumping volume of the heart-lung machine is gradually increased. Note the passive and parallel increase in MCA flow velocity indicating loss of cerebral autoregulation. *E* Minor cardiopulmonary perfusion at the end of the open heart intervention with spontaneous irregular myocardial activities (= systolic peaks). *F* Irregular heart beats (left part) are followed by frequent and regular myocardial actions (right part) due to stimulation with a pacemaker (arrow = start of the pacemaker)

flow velocities were only slightly affected by hypothermia or during the start of extracorporeal circulation, and were not affected by medium-sized extracranial carotid lesions in two patients. Surprisingly, reduced hemispheric flow velocities could not be recorded in two patients during the operation although severe postoperative encephalopathy was present. These findings, however, may in part be explained by accidental *hyper*perfusion of the brain. During intraoperative transcranial Doppler monitoring, Lundar *et al.* (1985) could observe various kinds of flow impairment. While initially *hyper*perfusion of the brain was a common finding, a complete loss of cerebral autoregulation was found during the subsequent phase of the operative procedure. These findings may have considerable clinical impact but further pathophysiological insights are necessary *before* the establishment of new treatment protocols.

In cardiopulmonary bypass patients, intraoperative monitoring of MCA flow velocity provides an ideal opportunity for testing the brain-protective potentials of various regimens in order to increase the tolerable MCA flow velocity reduction. However, such studies have not yet been carried out.

Transcranial Doppler Monitoring During Carotid Endarterectomy

This kind of monitoring may aid the vascular surgeon when he must decide on the security of carotid clamping. The need for a shunt, which has its own intrinsic morbidity (Ferguson 1982) can easily be evaluated. During tentative clamping of the carotid arteries, the severity of flow velocity drop will inform the surgeon whether this procedure will be critical or not. Illustrative effects of extracranial carotid clamping, shunting or flooding on the intracranial blood flow velocity are summarized in Fig. 3.

It is of particular importance that the effects of preoperative, tentative, manual compression of the common carotid artery on the MCA blood flow are in fact predictive of the intraoperative events during cross-clamping of the exposed carotid bifurcation. In a recent study from our group (Edelmann *et al.* 1985), a close relationship between preoperative and intraoperative MCA flow velocity reduction was evident. Other workers in this field, however, have not found such a close correlation (Gosling 1985, personal communication).

During a pre-, intra- and postoperative study on 35 patients with carotid endarterectomy a widely varying degree of flow velocity reduction within the MCA could be recorded. From the author's own experience, a time-mean flow velocity drop of less than 0.8 kHz Doppler shift (or of two thirds of the preclamping values in relative terms) obviously does not not require a shunt. None of these patients revealed any postoperative neurological deficit despite a 25–45 minute clamping period. From these findings a preliminary restriction of shunting procedures to patients with more severe

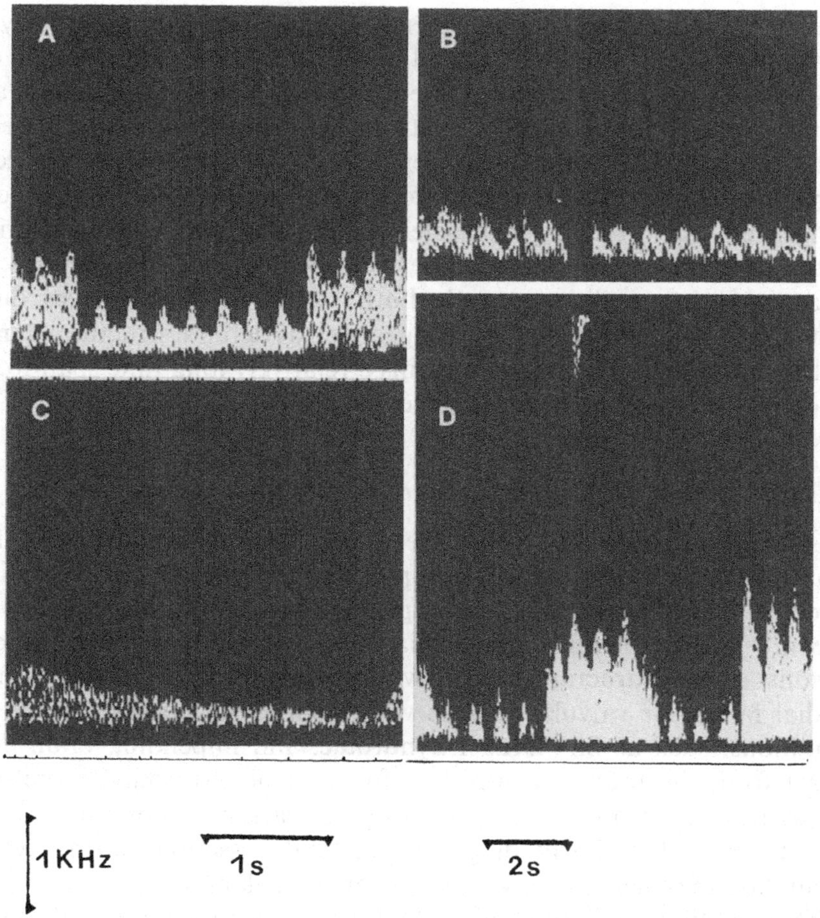

Fig. 3. Various effects of manipulation at the carotid bifurcation on MCA blood flow velocity during carotid endarterectomy. *A* Back-flow via the extracranial ICA leads to severe reduction of MCA flow velocity. *B* Back-flow via the extracranial ICA during one cardiac circle leads to reversal of blood flow (= downward deflection of the flow signal) within the stem of the MCA. *C* Manipulations at the carotid sinus lead to severe bradycardia (22 beats/min). However, diastolic blood velocity is maintained due to sufficient autoregulatory capacities. *D* During insertion of an indwelling shunt, periodic interruptions of MCA blood flow could be observed which paralleled thoracic excursions due to artificial ventilation. The surgeon became aware of this phenomenon only due to the TCD monitoring. Lack of diastolic blood flow during the phases with flow depression lead to the assumption of a valve mechanism within the shunt. In fact, during inspiration, the mouth of the shunt came into transient contact with the inner wall of the kinked ICA and was partially blocked

flow impairment during clamping seems to be justified. Retrospectively, the above-mentioned "threshold" would have lead to a shunt insertion in only 15% of the cases in our cohort (Edelmann *et al.* 1985). Presumably, a far more restricted subpopulation of patients definitely requires an indwelling shunt, but sufficient clinical experience is still lacking in order to define more precisely the critical border zone of an intolerable flow reduction (Ringelstein *et al.* 1985 b, Ringelstein 1986). Doppler monitoring is of particular interest in the surveillance of cerebrovascular interventions. The ultrasound abnormalities precede both functional disturbances during electrophysiological neuromonitoring as well as definite structural damage of the brain tissue. There thus remains a relatively long time span to take action to prevent permanent damage.

Transcranial Flow Veloctiy Monitoring During Intensive Care

This application of TCD is a very wide but still unexplored field. Monitoring may be informative and presumably beneficial for the patient's outcome in subarachnoid hemorrhage, high-pressure hydrocephalus, low-pressure hydrocephalus, intracranial pressure elevation due to other reasons, severe extracranial occlusive disease with low-flow states, myocardial failure or valvular disease with insufficient cardiac output, rare conditions, such as Shy-Drager-Syndrome, and impending brain death. Apart from the therapy-controlling function of ultrasound monitoring, deeper insights into the pathophysiology of various abnormal conditions may be provided. Early diagnosis of total cessation of the cerebral circulation may help to select donors for transplantation.

Due to still very limited clinical experience with transcranial Doppler monitoring, the author has confined himself to the following applications: 1. Monitoring of MCA blood flow during increased ICP, 2. Impending brain death, and 3. Intermittent monitoring of cerebral flow velocities during the spasm phase following subarachoid hemorrhage.

Fig. 4. Intermittent monitoring of MCA flow velocity following head trauma. *A* Initially (= day 1), the comatose patient showed normal MCA flow velocities. *B* During the following two days (= 2/3), hyperfusion occurred although PCO_2 was kept constant and within normal range. Intracranial pressure was also in normal limits (approx. 5–10 mm Hg). *C/D* On the fourth day, however, a sinusoid fluctuation of MCA flow velocities was recorded which paralleled ventilation-dependent alterations of intracranial pressure (*ICP*). This finding indicated loss of cerebral autoregulation. The flow velocities and the autoregulatory capacity normalized within the following week. However, the patient remained in a vegetative state

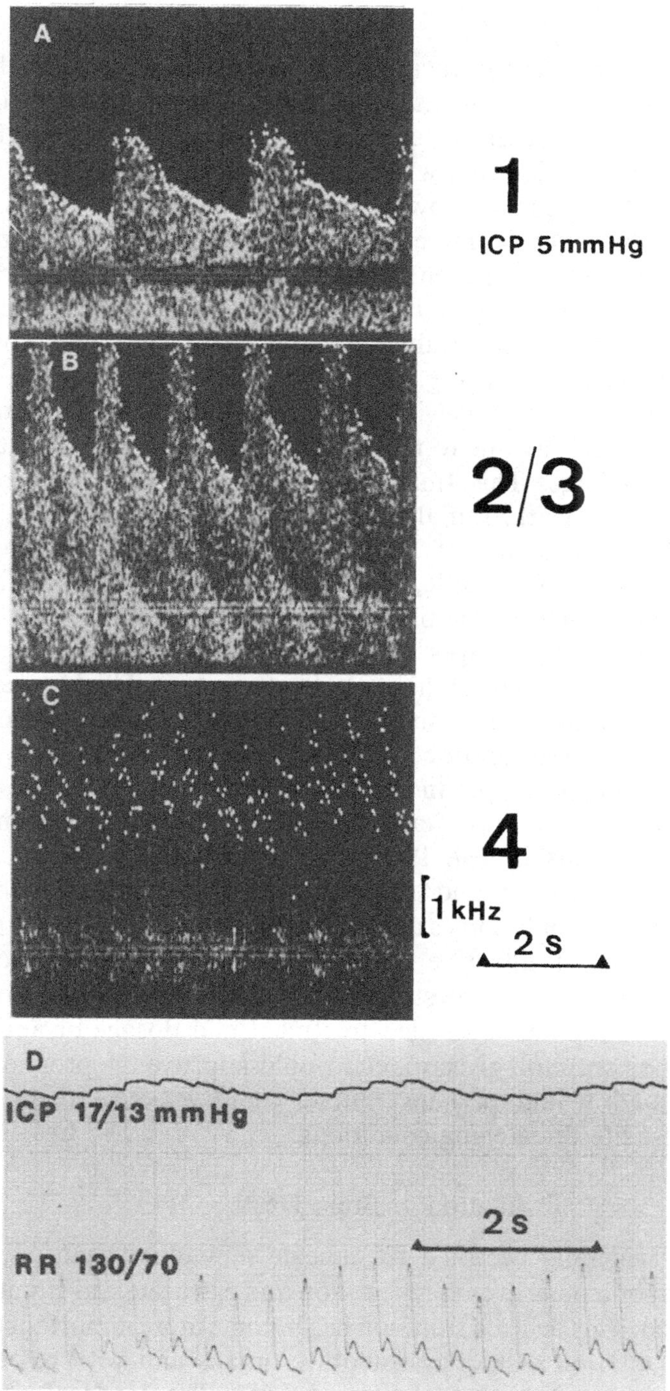
A
B
C
D
1
ICP 5 mmHg
2/3
4
1 kHz
2 s
ICP 17/13 mmHg
2 s
RR 130/70

Increasing Intracranial Pressure

A close relationship between intracranial pressure (ICP) on the one hand and MCA mean flow velocity or the shape of the flow profile on the other has not yet been demonstrated convincingly. However, the author's observations in several cases allow for some general remarks about the changes of MCA flow signals following ICP elevation. In some cases with head trauma, flow velocity was increased immediately after the *injury of the head*, lasting for several days or even weeks. During this period, intracranial pressure was only slightly elevated, if at all. The prognosis in these patients turned out to be dubious and resulted in a vegetative state in two out of three. An example is shown in Fig. 4. The ultrasound findings were quite different in another five patients with a severe increase of the intracranial pressure on the second day due to massive brain swelling with or without intracranial hemorrhage. This finally led to cessation of the cerebral circulation and brain death. Initially, a hyperperfusion profile (*i.e.*, high velocities, decrease of pulsatility of the signal) was also recorded but rapidly changed to an increasingly pulsatile, high-resistance flow profile and finally to a to-and-fro movement of the blood column (see Fig. 5).

One of the major disadvantages of this indirect, ultrasound approach to the evaluation of ICP is that pCO_2 has to be kept constant. This is necessary in order to obtain information on those hemodynamic changes merely induced by vasoparalysis and/or brain swelling and to exclude flow acceleration due to hypercapnia-induced vasodilatation.

Recently, Aaslid *et al.* have extracted a new parameter from the ultrasound profiles (Aaslid *et al.* 1985) which is highly indicative of the cerebral perfusion pressure and thus of the momentary intracranial pressure. If this approach becomes accepted, it would be of utmost interest for the large group of intensive care patients with ICP elevation in neurosurgery, neurology and anesthesiology. Presumably, a monitoring-based as well as computer-controlled treatment and dosage of anti-ICP substances such as sorbitol, glycerol, etc. would improve the prognosis of these patients and would perhaps initiate more effective therapeutic regimens in these life-threatening conditions.

Evaluation of Brain Death

Brain death is generally accepted to indicate individual death, *i.e.*, an irreversibly fatal outcome, even if respiration and extracerebral circulation are still preserved. This delicate situation has become more important in the light of transplantation of kidneys or other organs and with respect to ethical limitations of intensive care measurements. From a legal point of view (in the FRG), aortography is not allowed for merely diagnostic purposes in patients with presumed brain death. Therefore, angiography

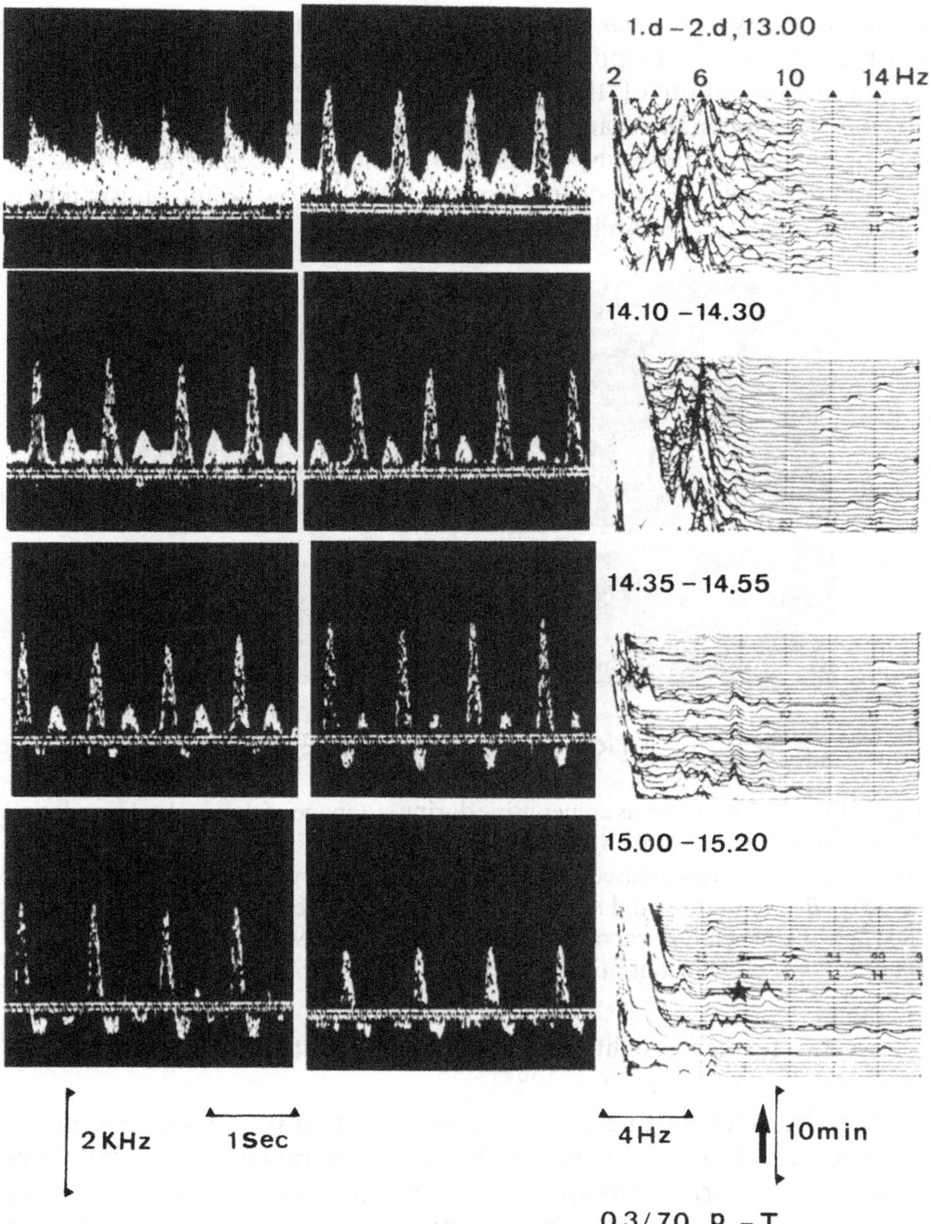

Fig. 5. Cessation of cerebral blood flow and brain death due to intracranial hemorrhage. *Left side*: The gradual development of a reverbaratory blood flow within the MCA is recorded in six steps over a period of two days. *Right side*: At the same time, EEG power spectrum deteriorated and showed isoelectricity as soon as the movement of the blood column became bidirectional. (Numbers indicate time p.m. on the second day)

cannot regulary be used as a quick diagnostic instrument in this condition. On the other hand, Doppler ultrasound is absolutely noninvasive when diagnosing cessation of the intracerebral circulation, but the findings strongly depend on the examiner's personal experience and can only poorly be documented. This is why ultrasound cannot be accepted as a standard method to diagnose brain death. However, MCA flow monitoring can be a valuable ancillary method for the evaluation of the patient's state and

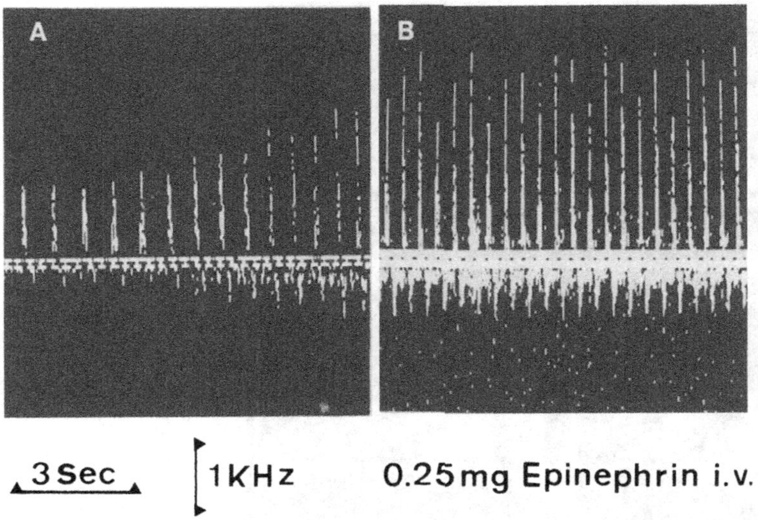

Fig. 6. Effect of intravenous epinephrine during stoppage of the cerebral circulation (same patient as in Fig. 5). *A* Immediately with the beginning of the injection, the cardiac ejection rate increased considerably, indicated by an increase in MCA flow velocity. *B* Two to threefold increase of MCA flow velocity (or perfusion pressure) did not overwhelm intracranial pressure and the MCA blood column was continuously rejected in the periphery

allows for further insights into the complex pathophysiological events during agonia (Ferbert *et al.* 1985).

The characteristic and diagnostic phenomenon is an oscillating movement of the blood column within the extracranial and/or the large intracranial arteries ("to-and-fro movement", Yoneda *et al.* 1974; see Fig. 5). Depending on the cardiac output, the flow profiles may be very sharp and pulsatile or, quite contrary, may be damped with sluggish acceleration and deceleration of the blood column. A reflux phenomenon during late systole following antegrade injection of the blood into the vascular tree is essential for the diagnosis in every case. Transcranial Doppler monitoring findings showing the gradual development of the circulatory arrest within the brain are documented in Fig. 5.

Immediately after the manifestation of the intracranial circulatory cessation, application of epinephrine in the same patient led to a severe increase of the heart ejection rate but systemic arterial pressure did not overcome the intracranial pressure. Cerebral perfusion pressure was still negative and blood flow in the basal arteries remained reverberaroty (Fig. 6).

Monitoring of Vasospasm Following Subarachnoid Hemorrhage

In the author's opinion, the preclinical noninvasive detection of vasospasm due to subarachnoid hemorrhage is the most remarkable progress in this field during the last years with particular respect to the therapeutic implications. Calcium-antagonists have been found to be effective in this problematic conditition. However, due to side-effects, a *selective* application of calcium antagonists for prevention of severe vasospasm and spasm-induced infarctions is mandatory. This selectiveness can now be realized with the help of TCD (Aaslid *et al.* 1982, 1984).

Elevated flow velocities in the MCA following subarachnoid hemorrhage have been categorized both by Seiler (see chapter 8, p. 125) and by Harders (see chapter 9, p. 138).

On admission of patients with acute subarachnoid hemorrhage, Seiler and co-workers (1985) found a direct correlation between the increase of the MCA flow velocities during TCD and the clinical state of the patients according to the Hunt and Hess scale. Increasing flow velocities paralleled the deterioration of the patient during the following days.

The effect of the TCD-controlled application of nimodipine in subarachnoid hemorrhage is a marked reduction of severe spasms as is indicated by lower flow velocities within the affected basal artery. These findings have been shown independently by several groups (Harders *et al.* 1985, Seiler *et al.* 1985).

Intermittent velocity monitoring for the detection of vasospasm due to subarachnoid hemorrhage should be carried out twice a day (or at least daily) in order to detect spasm development in a preclinical phase allowing therapeutic measures to be preventive.

Multimodal Approaches

During severe reduction or even cessation of blood flow within the cerebral arteries, the exact sequence of events and their precise time relationship are still unknown. Multimodal monitorings, including various electrophysiological as well as circulatory parameters are a new and attractive way of studying the nervous tissue function and blood supply both simultaneously and absolutely on-line. As far as is known, such studies have not yet been published apart from a personal observation in a patient with developing brain death due to severe intracerebral hemorrhage. The simultaneous recordings of the EEG power spectrum and the MCA flow profiles were paralleled in Fig. 5. When the pathognomic phenomenon of cerebral flow cessation, *i.e.*, the to-and-fro movement of the blood column occurred, the EEG became isoelectric. During the preceeding stage with marked pulsatility of the flow profile due to severely increased peripheral vascular resistance, a burst suppression pattern was prominent in the EEG.

Further studies are under way including transcranial Doppler flow measurement within the MCA together with hemispheric monitoring of SEP and repetitive motor pathway stimulations during intraoperative carotid clamping, with and without medical brain protection.

Conclusions

This report, although still anecdotal in most parts, gives an interim overview of the potentials of TCD as a monitoring instrument in neurology, neurosurgery and cardiovascular interventions. Some applications of TCD have still been realized by a limited number of workers in the field of neurosonology whereas others only seem to be proposals for the future. At present, monitoring techniques in clinical neurosciences are rapidly progressing and new pathophysiological knowledge accumulates.

Up to now, the practical usefulness of TCD monitoring has predominantly been shown during carotid endarterectomy with respect to the shunting problem, and during open heart surgery for control of adequate arterial blood supply and analysis of cerebral autoregulation (Ringelstein *et al.* 1985 a, von Reutern *et al.* 1985, Lundar *et al.* 1985). It seems very attractive for neurosonologists to elicit what is really going on in the brain vessels when the surgeon manipulates at the supraaortic arteries or at the heart itself. Presumably, unexpected Doppler findings will lead to the abolishment of seemingly necessary—but in fact useless or even dangerous—conventions such as superfluous insertion of a shunt during carotid endarterectomy. Another aim is the establishment of more adequate regimens during cardiopulmonary bypassing. In the near future, typical TCD flow patterns associated with adverse neurological outcomes must be defined so that they can promptly be recognized during intensive care surveillance or intraoperatively *before* permanent damage occurs. To be effective, monitors must give early warning of potentially dangerous situations.

Prospectively, further applications of monitoring will deliver new and exciting insights into the physiology and pathophysiology of cerebral circulation by monitoring of cerebral blood flow during epileptic seizures and other kinds of syncopes, monitoring of MCA blood flow during extreme changes of body position, TCD monitoring during neuroradiological interventions such as balloon occlusions, embolization of A-V shunts or intra-arterial fibrinolysis, and monitoring for antigravity influences on cardiovascular parameters during research in space (see Pourcelot *et al.* 1984).

This list, of course, is incomplete and just mentions only a few of the most obvious possibilities.

References

Aaslid R, Markwalder T, Nornes H (1982) Noninvasive transcranial Doppler ultrasound recording of flow velocity in basal arteries. J Neurosurg 57: 769–774

Aaslid R, Huber P, Nornes H (1984) Evaluation of cerebrovascular spasm with transcranial Doppler ultrasound. J Neurosurg 60: 37–41

Aaslid R, Lundar T, Lindegaard K-F, Nornes H (1985) Estimation of cerebral perfusion pressure from arterial blood pressure and transcanial Doppler recordings. In: Teasdale G, Brock M (eds) Intracranial pressure 6. Springer, Berlin Heidelberg New York

Edelmann M, Richert F, Messmer B, Ringelstein EB (1985) Monitoring of middle cerebral artery blood flow velocity during carotid endarterectomy with the aid of transcranial Doppler sonography. In: Diagnostic ultrasound in neurology, neurosurgery and neuropediatrics. Satellite symposium of the XIIIth world congress of neurology, Aachen, August 30–September 1, 1985

Ferbert A, Buchner H, Wulfinghoff F, Korbmacher G, Ringelstein EB, Hacke W (1986) Neurophysiological and neurosonological findings in isolated brain stem death. In: Clinical problems of brain stem disorders. Satellite symposium of the XIIIth world congress of neurology, Hamburg, August 31–September 1, 1985, Thieme, Stuttgart, New York

Ferguson (1982) Intra-operative monitoring and internal shunts: Are they necessary in carotid endarterectomy? Stroke 13: 3, 287–289

Furlan AJ, Breuer A (1984) Central nervous system complications of open heart surgery. Stroke 15: 912–915

Grosse W, Matentzoglu S, Wulfinghoff F, Ringelstein EB, (1985) The transcranial Doppler approach to vasomotor reactivity. In: Diagnostic ultrasound in neurology, neurosurgery and neuropediatrics. Satellite symposium of the XIIIth world congress and neurology, Aachen, August 30–September 1

Hacke W (1985) Neuromonitoring. J Neurol 232: 125–133

Harders A, Hilger Y, Gilsbach J (1985) Transcranial Doppler sonography. Evaluation of hemodynamic changes in the circle of Willis after spontaneous subarachnoid hemorrhage due to vasospasm. In: Diagnostic ultrasound in neurology, neurosurgery and neuropediatrics. Satellite symposium of the XIIIth world congress of neurology, Aachen, August 30–September 1, 1985

Henriksen L, Hjems E, Lindeburgh T (1983) Brain hyperperfusion during cardiac operations: Cerebral blood flow measured in man by intra-arterial injection of Xenon 133: Evidence suggestive of intraoperative microembolism. Thorac Cardiovasc Surg 86: 202–211

Jacobs LA, Brinkman SD, Morrell RM, Shirley JG, Ganji S (1983) Long-latency somatosensory evoked potentials during carotid endarterectomy. Amer Surg 49: 338–344

Lundar T, Lindegaard K-F, Fröysaker T, Aaslid R, Wiberg J, Nornes H (1985) Cerebral perfusion during nonpulsatile cardiopulmonary bypass. Ann Thorac Surg 40: 144–148

Markand ON, Dilley RS, Moorthy SS, Warren Jr C (1984) Monitoring of somatosensory evoked responses during carotid endarterectomy. Arch Neurol 41: 375–378

Mickey B, Vorstrup S, Voldby B, Lindewald H, Harmsen A, Lassen NA (1984) Serial measurement of regional cerebral blood flow in patients with SAH using 133Xe inhalation and emission computerized tomography. J Neurosurg 60: 916–922

Obrist WD, Gennarelli TA, Segawa H, Dolinskas CA, Langfitt TW (1979) Relation of cerebral blood flow to neurological status and outcome in head-injured patients. J Neurosurg 51: 292–300

Pourcelot L, Arbeille Ph, Pottier JM, Patat F, Mignier P, Guell A, Charib C (1984) Ultrasonic study of early cardiovascular adaptation to zero gravitiy. Proc. 2nd European symposium on life science and research in space, Porz Wahn, Germany, June 4–6, 1984

von Reutern GM, Hetzel A, Arnolds B, Schlosser V (1985) Flow velocity in the middle cerebral artery during heart surgery with cardiopulmonary bypass. In: Diagnostic ultrasound in neurology, neurosurgery and nauropediatrics. Satellite symposium of the XIIIth world congress of neurology, Aachen, August 30–September 1, 1985

Ries F, Tsuda Y, Hartmann A, Lagreze H, Seiler R (1985) Correlation of rCBF measurement and transcranial Doppler sonography during normo- and hypocapnia in patients with CVD and normals. In: Diagnostic ultrasound in neurology, neurosurgery and neuropediatrics. Satellite symposium of the XIIIth world congress of neurology, Aachen, August 30–September 1, 1985

Ringelstein EB, Grosse W, Matenzoglu S (1985 a) The transcranial Doppler approach to vasomotor reserve. In: Cerebrovascular ultrasound. International symposium, Seattle, Washington, May 13–15, 1985

Ringelstein EB, Richert F, Bardos S, Minale C, Alsukun M, Zeplin H, Schöndube F, Zeumer H, Messmer B (1985 b) Transkraniell-sonographisches Monitoring des Blutflusses der A. cerebri media während rekanalisierender Operationen an der extrakraniellen A. carotis interna. Nervenarzt 56: 423–430

Ringelstein EB, Wulfinghoff F, Brückmann H, Zeumer H, Hacke W, Buchner H (1986 c) Transcranial Doppler sonography as a non-invasive guide for the transvascular treatment of an inoperable basilar-artery aneurysm. Neurol Res 7: (in press)

Ringelstein EB, Edelmann M, Richert F, Minale C, Bardos S, Messmer B (1987) Transcranial Doppler monitoring of medial cerebral artery flow velocity during carotid endarterectomy. J Neurol (in press)

Seiler RW, Grolimund P, Zurbrügg HR, Reulen H-J (1985) Evaluation of the efficacy of nimodipine for the prevention of cerebral vasospasm following subarachnoid hemorrhage by transcranial Doppler sonography. In: Diagnostic ultrasound in neurology, neurosurgery and neuropediatrics. Satellite symposium of the XIIIth world congress of neurology, Aachen, August 30–September 1, 1985

Sundt TM, Sharbrough FW, Piepgras DG, Kearns TP, Messick JM, O'Fallon WM (1981) Correlation of cerebral blood flow and electroencephalographic changes during carotid endarterectomy. Mayo Clin Proc 56: 533–543

Yoneda YS, Nishimoto A, Nukada T (1974) To-and-fro movement and external escape of carotid arterial blood in brain death cases. A Doppler ultrasonic study. Stroke 5: 707–713

Author's address: Dr. E. B. Ringelstein, Department of Neurology, RWTH University, Pauwelstrasse, D-5100 Aachen, Federal Republic of Germany.

11. Transcranial Doppler in the Study of Cerebral Perfusion During Cardiopulmonary Bypass

T. Lundar

Studies of the cerebral circulation during cardiopulmonary bypass (CPB) procedures have been severely hampered by methodological difficulties. Compared with the large numbers of cardiac operations performed each year, knowledge on cerebral perfusion has been remarkably scarce, especially since cerebral damage remains a major and devastating complication of cardiac surgery [5]. Early experimental studies using electromagnetic carotid artery flowmetry, indicated that carotid flow fluctuated passively with flow from the heart-lung machine during nonpulsatile cardiopulmonary bypass [4, 7].

Early clinical studies were based on the coupling of cerebral flow and metabolism, and indirect estimation of cerebral blood flow from observed cerebral arteriovenous differences ($AVDO_7$) [4]. Recent animal studies have, however, indicated that the coupling of cerebral blood flow and metabolism is lost during nonpulsatile CPB [3]. Indirect estimation of cerebral blood flow (CBF) from $AVDO_2$. therefore does not seem to be justified under these circumstances. A few clinical reports on CBF during CPB based on Xenon washout techniques, have been presented during the last years. The results are conflicting: Henriksen and co-workers reported markedly enhanced perfusion during nonpulsatile CPB [8], while Govier *et al.* [6] found a clear reduction of the cerebral circulation during CPB. The regimens for cardiopulmonary bypass were not identical, yet the discrepancies seem difficult to explain. A small clinical series of electromagnetically recorded internal carotid artery (ICA) flowmetry throughout cardiopulmonary bypass, confirmed the results of Henriksen *et al.*—increased cerebral perfusion during moderately hypothermic, nonpulsatile CPB [2].

Assessment of the middle cerebral artery (MCA) flow velocity by the new, noninvasive transcranial Doppler (TCD) technique [1], offers new opportunities for studies of cerebral circulation. The TCD method has proved to be of value in the management of patients with subarachnoid hemorrhage [2] as well as patients with precerebral occlusive artery disease [10].

The diameter of the proximal MCA is assumed to be relatively constant [9, 16] as regulation of cerebrovascular resistance acts on the arteriolar level,

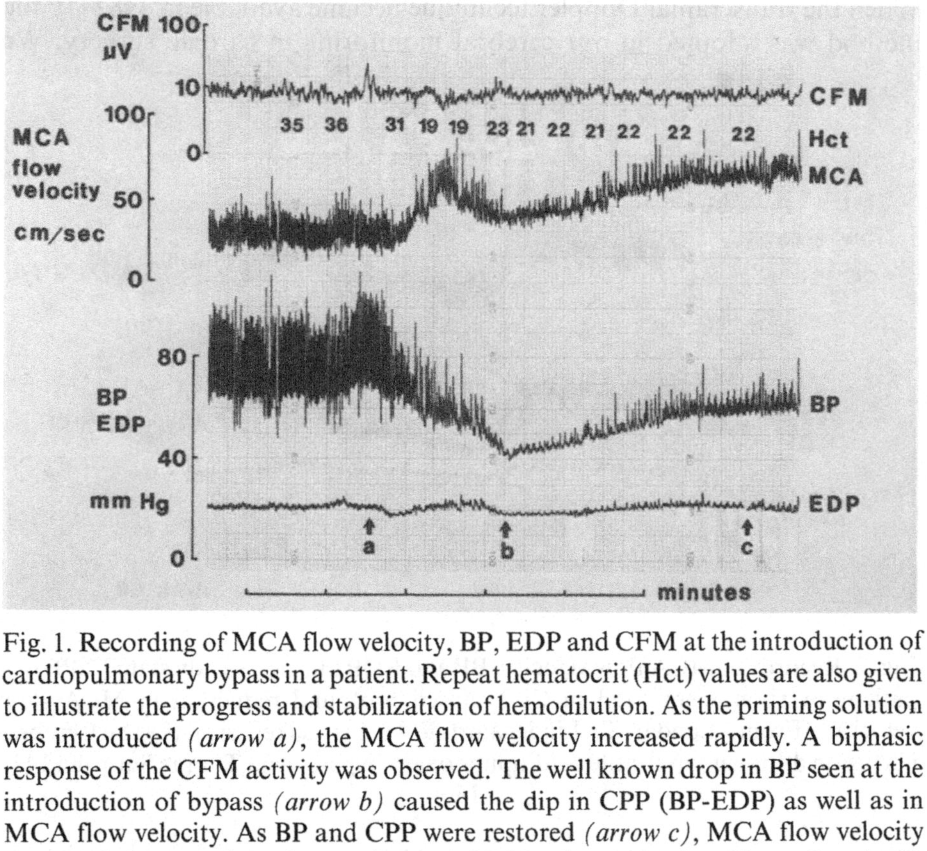

Fig. 1. Recording of MCA flow velocity, BP, EDP and CFM at the introduction of cardiopulmonary bypass in a patient. Repeat hematocrit (Hct) values are also given to illustrate the progress and stabilization of hemodilution. As the priming solution was introduced *(arrow a)*, the MCA flow velocity increased rapidly. A biphasic response of the CFM activity was observed. The well known drop in BP seen at the introduction of bypass *(arrow b)* caused the dip in CPP (BP-EDP) as well as in MCA flow velocity. As BP and CPP were restored *(arrow c)*, MCA flow velocity once again increased, to about twice the initial (prebypass) value. [From: Lundar T, Lindegaard K-F, Frøysaker T, *et al* (1985) Cerebral perfusion during nonpulsatile cardiopulmonary bypass. Ann Thorac Surg 40: 144–150]

both in autoregulation of cerebral blood flow during changes in cerebral perfusion pressure (CPP = mean arterial blood pressure–mean intracranial pressure) as well as during carbon dioxide induced changes in the cerebral perfusion. Comparative observations on MCA flow velocity and electromagnetically recorded ICA flow have revealed that changes in MCA flow velocity reflect concomitant changes in cerebral perfusion. A recent study reports the effect of changes in pCO_2 on MCA flow velocity in healthy volunteers [15]. The demonstrated classic CO_2 effect on cerebral circulation further supports that observed changes in MCA flow velocities are related to similar changes in MCA volume flow.

Transcranial Doppler Recording During Cardiac Surgery

When the transcranial Doppler technique became available in 1982 [1], the method was adopted in our cerebral monitoring in cardiac surgery. We

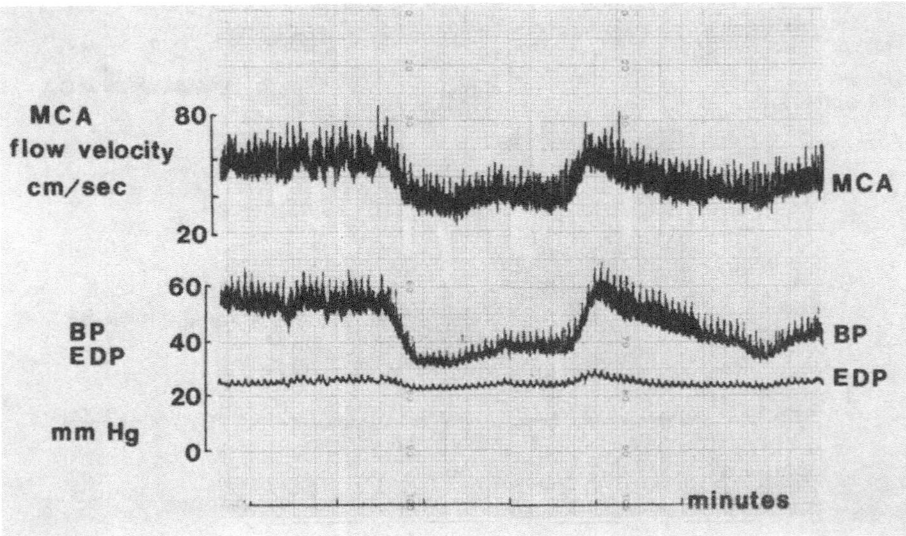

Fig. 2. Records of MCA flow velocity, BP and EDP during "steady state" CPB in a patient. A spontaneous fall in CPP caused profound reduction in MCA flow velocity. [From: Lundar T, Lindegaard K-F, Frøysaker *et al* (1985) Cerebral perfusion during nonpulsatile cardiopulmonary bypass. Ann Thorac Surg. 40: 144–150]

have, for several years, performed extensive cerebral monitoring in highly selected cases, deemed to be at high risk for cerebral complications during and after cardiac surgery. Such risk factors include previous stroke, anticipated extracorporeal perfusion time exceeding 120 minutes, multiple valvular replacement, combined valvular replacement and aortocoronary bypass procedures, aortic arch aneurysmectomies and revalvular replacements.

The monitoring includes recording of arterial blood pressure (BP), central venous pressure (CVP) and epidural intracranial pressure (EDP). A minitransducer is implanted through a burrhole in the right frontal region in advance of the surgical procedure [11]. Cerebral electrical activity is recorded by a cerebral function monitor (CFM).

Continuous recording of MCA flow velocity throughout CPB, generally demonstrated markedly increased flow velocities [14]. As the diameter of the MCA is unknown in the individual patient, comparison of the flow velocities between the patients has no meaning. Compared with the flow velocity recorded during the last 5 minutes before CPB (prebypass level),

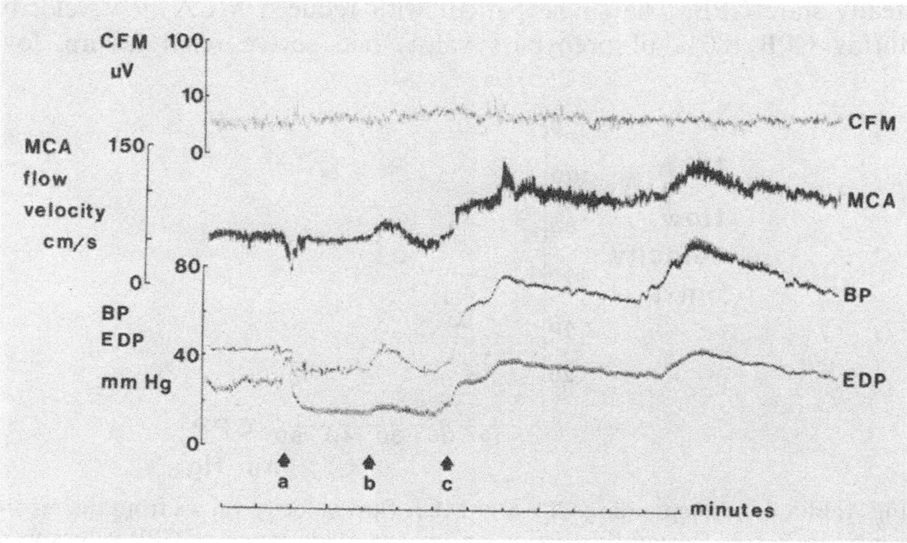

Fig. 3. Records of BP, EDP, MCA flow velocity and CFM activity during an 18-minute period of cardiopulmonary bypass in a patient. From a low CPP state of 23 mm Hg, a short-term obstruction of the venous return caused an abrupt increase in the central venous pressure and EDP, and a CPP reduction to about 5 mm Hg *(arrow a)*. The corresponding fall in MCA flow velocity is clearly seen. Administration of 1 mg metaraminol *(arrow b)* and increased pump flow from 1.8 to 2.1 l/min/m^2 *(arrow c)* caused marked increase in CPP and MCA flow velocity. The marked changes in the intracranial pressure (EDP) are clearly demonstrated. [From: Lundar T, Lindegaard K-F, Frøysaker T *et al* (1985) Dissocation between cerebral autoregulation and CO_2 reactivity during non-pulsatile cardiopulmonary bypass. Ann Thorac Surg 40: 582–587]

changes in percentual value of prebypass level will reflect concomitant changes in cerebral perfusion in the individual patient.

At the introduction of CPB, MCA flow velocities increased in spite of an abrupt reduction in the cerebral perfusion pressure (CPP = BP-EDP) at the inception of the extracorporeal perfusion. Introduction of the priming solution caused, however, concomitant rapid hemodilution, resulting in hematocrit values of about half of prebypass level. At this point, CPP was reduced to below 30 mm Hg for a minute or two. This lowest CPP "dip" caused a temporary reduction of the increased MCA flow velocity after the initial increase, before MCA flow velocity was stabilized at 150–300% of the individual prebypass value [14]. These initial events are illustrated in Fig. 1, demonstrating the increase in MCA flow velocity at introduction of CPB, influenced by rapid changes in CPP and hematocrit.

The first series of 11 patients with MCA flow velocity monitoring during CPB [14], revealed enhanced flow velocities in 10 out of 11 patients during steady state CPB. The single patient with reduced MCA flow velocity during CPB (80% of prebypass value) had severe renal failure, low

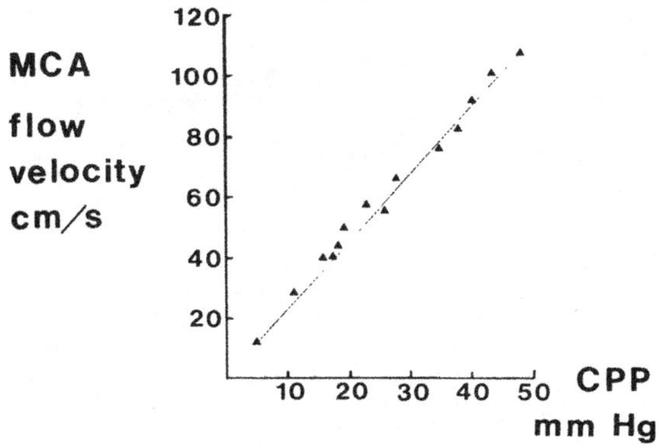

Fig. 4. Plot of corresponding CPP and MCA flow velocity values from the record period in Fig. 3. During this period an unusual wide range of CPP values were observed (5–48 mm Hg). The linear relationship indicates a pressure passive, non-autoregulatory situation. [From: Lundar T, Lindegaard K-F, Frøysaker T, *et al* (1985) Dissociation between cerebral autoregulation and CO_2 reactivity during nonpulsatile cardiopulmonary bypass. Ann Thorac Surg 40: 582–587]

hematocrit before operation, and subsequently less hemodilution at the introduction of CPB.

In all the 10 patients where MCA flow velocity recording was continued during the first 15 minutes after termination of CPB, flow velocities were still moderately to markedly increased compared to prebypass values [14].

Cerebral Autoregulation During CPB

Although MCA flow velocities were generally increased during nonpulsatile CPB, the flow velocities varied in a pressure passive manner with changing CPP. Examples are given in Figs. 2 and 3, where the influence of changes in CPP on MCA flow velocity are clearly seen. These observations were obtained during periods with constant temperature, hematocrit and $PaCO_2$. A plot of the relationship between CPP and MCA flow velocity from Fig. 3, is presented in Fig. 4, clearly indicating that the cerebral autoregulation was not operative.

CO_2-Reactivity Tests

The influence of changes in $PaCO_2$ on MCA flow velocity can be tested during CPB. Increasing gas flow to the membrane oxygenator of the heart-lung machine, causes instant reduction of $PaCO_2$—and reduction of MCA flow velocity from one steady state level to another. The recording of MCA

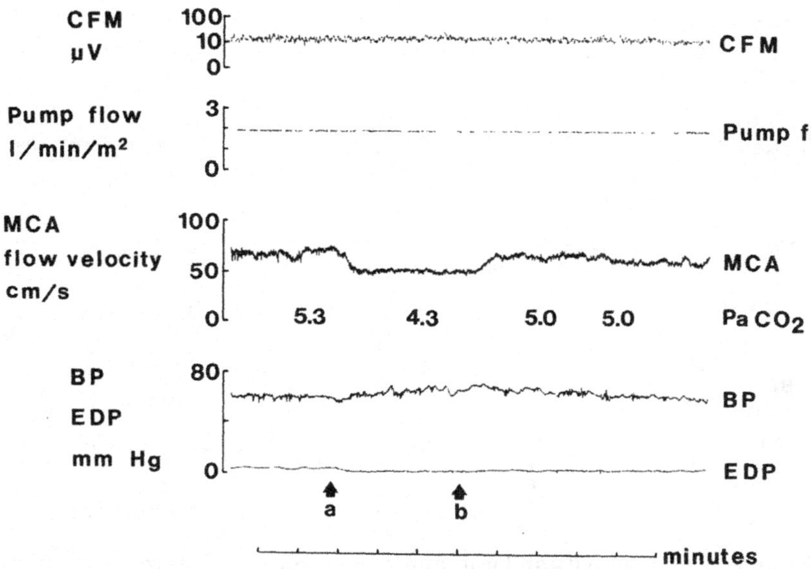

Fig. 5. Recording of CFM, pump flow, MCA flow velocity, BP and EDP during a CO_2 reactivity test. $PaCO_2$ was determined every 30 seconds. Gas flow to the membrane oxygenator was increased from 1.4 to 10.0 l/min *(arrow a)* and reversed from 10.0 to 1.4 l/min after 3 minutes *(arrow b)*. Preserved CO_2 reactivity is clearly demonstrated. [From: Lundar T, Lindegaard K-F, Frøysaker T, *et al* (1985) Dissociation between cerebral autoregulation and CO_2 reactivity during non-pulsatile cardiopulmonary bypass. Ann Thorac Surg 40: 582–587]

flow velocity, BP, EDP and CFM during a CO_2 reactivity test is presented in Fig. 5. The cerebral CO_2 reactivity is usually defined as per cent change in cerebral blood flow per mm Hg change in $PaCO_2$. In CO_2 reactivity tests using TCD technique, we have defined cerebral CO_2 reactivity as percent change in MCA flow velocity per mm Hg change in temperature corrected $PaCO_2$ [13]. During most CO_2 reactivity tests, a reduction of EDP caused by concomitant reduction in cerebral blood volume was observed (Fig. 6). This is a well known observation in neurosurgical practice, and another demonstration of the CO_2 effect upon the cerebral vasculature.

Studies of cerebral CO_2 reactivity in 5 patients during moderately hypothermic (28–32 °C), low flow (1.5 l/min/m [2] body surface), non-pulsatile cardiopulmonary bypass, demonstrated preserved CO_2 reactivity in all patients [13]. The CO_2 reactivities were in the range of 1.9 to 4.1% mm Hg [13], observed at CPP levels ranging from 28 to 60 mm Hg.

In one single patient, we have been able to record ICA flow and MCA

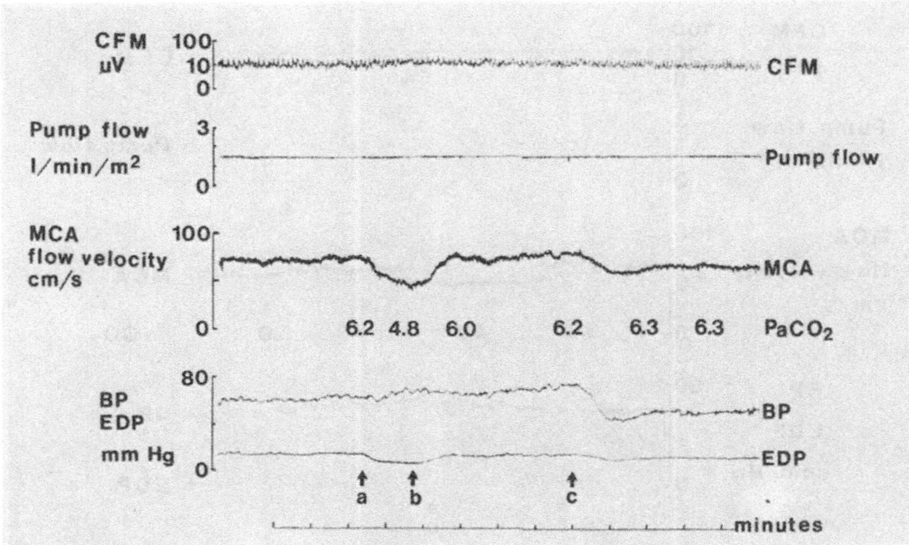

Fig. 6. Retained CO_2 reactivity and non-autoregulation. Gas flow to the membrane oxygenator was increased from 1.0 to 10.0 l/min *(arrow a)* and reversed from 10.0 to 1.0 l/min *(arrow b)*. A clear CO_2 response was observed in spite of an increase in CPP. Note the effect on EDP from the $PaCO_2$ reduction. Administration of 2.5 mg chlorpromazine *(arrow c)* caused a fall in CPP from 60 to 45 mm Hg and a reduced MCA flow velocity from 80 to 60 cm/sec. [From: Lundar T, Lindegaard K-F, Frøysaker T *et al* (1985) Dissociation between cerebral autoregulation and CO_2 reactivity during nonpulsatile cardiopulmonary bypass. Ann Thorac Surg 40: 582–587]

flow velocity simultaneously during cardiopulmonary bypass. This was in a patient who underwent ICA endarterectomy in advance of an aortacoronary bypass procedure [14]. The concomitant changes in electromagnetically recorded ICA flow and MCA flow velocity caused by changes in cerebral perfusion pressure during a 5-minute period, are demonstrated in Fig. 7.

The studies of MCA flow velocity during CPB demonstrate that the cerebral perfusion is enhanced during moderately hypothermic, non-pulsatile cardiopulmonary bypass. This increased cerebral perfusion is, however, dependent on the regimen for CPB, since changes in pump flow or variations in CPP resulting from fluctuations in BP and EDP, cause

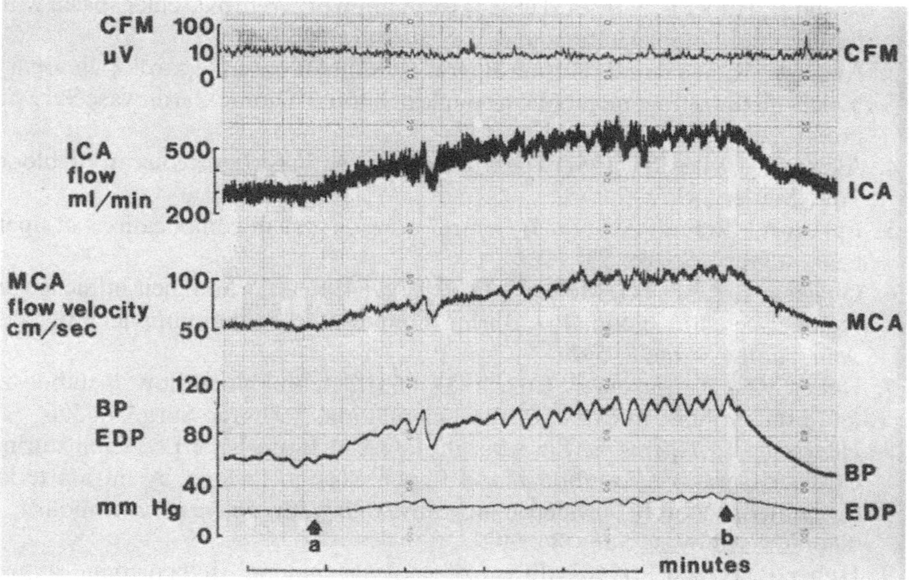

Fig. 7. Simultaneous recording of MCA flow velocity, ipsilateral internal carotid artery (ICA) flow, BP, EDP and CFM during established CPB in a patient. Increase in machine flow from 1.5 to 2.0 l/min/m^2 body surface *(arrow a)*, caused a marked increase in MCA flow velocity and ICA flow. Note the close relationship between the MCA flow velocity and the ICA flow changes. As machine flow was reduced from 2.0 to 1.5 l/min/m^2 body surface *(arrow b)*, subsequent reductions in CPP, MCA flow velocity and ICA flow were observed. During the increased machine flow, "vasomotor waves" in BP were seen. Concomitant changes in EDP, MCA flow velocity and ICA flow are also demonstrated. Temperature (28°C), hemodilution (Hct 24) and $PaCO_2$ (temperature corrected 38 mm Hg) were constant during the recording. [From: Lundar T, Lindegaard K-F, Frøysaker T *et al* (1985) Cerebral perfusion during nonpulsatile cardiopulmonary bypass. Ann Thorac Surg 40: 144–150]

concomitant changes in cerebral perfusion. The demonstrated preservation of cerebral CO_2 reactivity imply that, during nonpulsatile cardiopulmonary bypass, there is a dissociation between cerebral autoregulation and CO_2 reactivity.

Recording of MCA flow velocity by TCD technique appears to be a useful tool in research for optimal extracorporeal perfusion and brain protection during CPB in the future.

References

1. Aaslid R, Markwalder TM, Nornes H (1982) Noninvasive transcranial Doppler ultrasound recording of flow velocity in basal cerebral arteries. J Neurosurg 57: 769

2. Aaslid R, Huber P, Nornes H (1984) Evaluation of cerebrovascular spasm with transcranial Doppler ultrasound. J Neurosurg 60: 37
3. Andersen K, Waaben J, Husum B, *et al* (1986) Nonpulsatile cardiopulmonary bypass disrupts flow-metabolism couple in brain. J Thorac Cardiovasc Surg (in press)
4. Akeney J L, Viles PH (1961) The effect of total body perfusion on carotid blood flow. Surgery 49: 209
5. Furlan AJ, Breurer AC (1984) Central nervous system complications of open heart surgery. Stroke 15: 912
6. Govier AV, Reves JG, McKay RD, *et al* (1984) Factors and their influence on regional cerebral blood flow during nonpulsatile cardiopulmonary bypass. Ann Thorac Surg 38: 592
7. Halley MM, Reemtsma K, Creech O (1958) Cerebral blood flow, metabolism and brain volume in extracorporeal circulation. J Thorac Surg. 36: 506
8. Henriksen L, Hjelms E, Lindeburgh T (1983) Brain hyperperfusion during cardiac operations: cerebral blood flow measured in man by intra-arterial injection of xenon 133: evidence suggestive of intraoperative microembolism. J Thorac Cardiovasc Surg. 86: 202
9. Huber P, Handa J (1967) Effect of contrast material, hypercapnia, hyperventilation, hypertonic glucose and papaverine on the diameter of the cerebral arteries: angiographic determination in man. Invest Radiol 2: 17
10. Lindegaard K-F, Grolimund P, Bakke SJ, *et al* (1985) Assessment of intracranial hemodynamics in carotid artery disease by transcranial Doppler ultrasound. J Neurosurg 63: 890
11. Lundar T, Frøysaker T, Nornes H, Lilleaasen P (1982) Aspects of cerebral perfusion in open-heart surgery. Scand J Thorac Cardiovasc Surg 16: 217
12. Lundar T, Frøysaker T, Lindegaard K-F, *et al* (1985) Some observations on cerebral perfusion during cardiopulmonary bypass. Ann Thorac Surg 39: 318
13. Lundar T, Lindegaard K-F, Frøysaker T, *et al* (1985) Dissocation between cerebral autoregulation and CO_2 reactivity during nonpulsatile cardiopulmonary bypass. Ann Thorac Surg 40: 582
14. Lundar T, Lindegaard K-F, Frøysaker T, *et al* (1985) Cerebral perfusion during nonpulsatile cardiopulmonary bypass. Ann Thorac Surg 40: 144–150
15. Markwalder TM, Grolimund P, Seiler RW, *et al* (1984) Dependency of blood flow velocity in the middle cerebral artery on end-tidal carbon dioxide pressure—A transcranial ultrasound Doppler study. J Cereb Blood Flow Metab. 4: 368
16. Strandgaard S, Paulson OB (1984) Cerebral autoregulation. Stroke 15: 413
17. Wollman H, Stephen GW, Clement AJ, Danielson GK (1966) Cerebral blood flow in man during extracorporeal circulation. J Thorac Cardiovasc Surg 52: 558

Author's address: Dr. T. Lundar, Department of Neurosurgery, Rikshospitalet, N-0027 Oslo 1, Norway.

Subject Index

J. M. Gilsbach

Intraoperative Doppler Sonography in Neurosurgery

1983. 61 figures. X, 104 pages.
ISBN 3-211-81768-9

Fully illustrated with diagrams and Doppler curve traces, "Intraoperative Doppler Sonography in Neurosurgery" demonstrates how the surgeon can improve the technique and safety of his operations with this "intravascular eye". The surgeon will no longer be dependent upon deceptive external appearances. Surgical procedures can be controlled close to the vessel allowing for an immediate decision in operative surgery.
The principles of Doppler measurement and the equipment used are discussed in great detail with emphasis on normal and pathological findings in microanastomoses, aneurysms, and bypass operations.
Previously unpublished information about Doppler intraoperative measurement applied to cerebrovascular operations and experimental microvascular surgery is presented in detailed case studies.
An introductory explanation is also included.

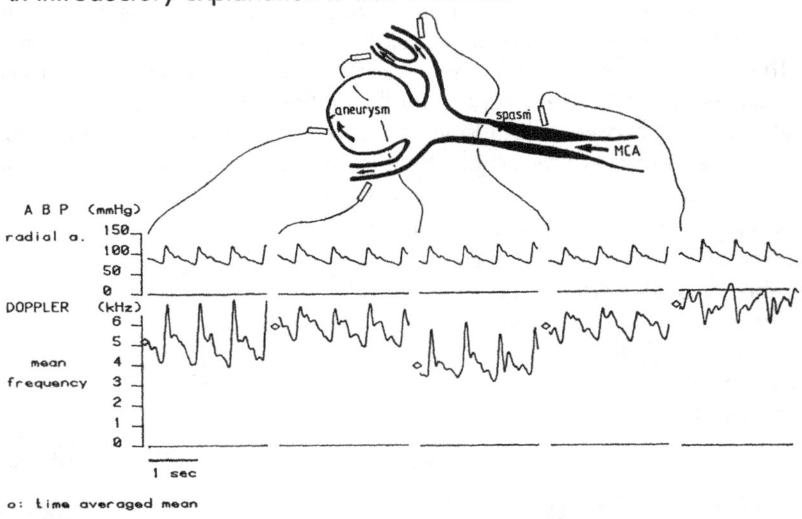

Springer-Verlag Wien New York

Made in the USA
Monee, IL
13 September 2026

62975222R00109